THE
Healing Benefits
OF
GARLIC

THE
Healing Benefits
OF
GARLIC

JOHN HEINERMAN, Ph.D.

WINGS BOOKS
New York

This 1995 edition is published by Wings Books, distributed by Random House Value Publishing, Inc., 201 East 50th Street, New York, New York 10022, by arrangement with Keats Publishing, Inc.

Random House
New York · Toronto · London · Sydney · Auckland
http://www.randomhouse.com/
Printed and bound in the United States of America

Library of Congress Cataloging–in–Publication Data

Heinerman, John.
    The healing benefits of garlic / John Heinerman.
        p. cm.
    Originally published: New Canaan, Conn., Keats, 1994.
    Includes index.
    ISBN 0-517-12444-0
    1. Garlic—Therapeutic use. 2. Garlic. 3. Cookery (Garlic)
I. Title.
RM666.G15H46   1995
615'.324324—dc20   94-47671
                                                CIP

8 7 6

To
The three best boys I ever knew—

Joseph and John Tipton of Plainview, Texas,
        and
Matthew Fountaine of Salt Lake City, Utah.

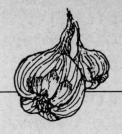

Contents

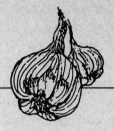

Introduction

IN THE beginning of 1992, I happened to phone the president of Keats Publishing, who told me that he was intending to do a book on garlic. I volunteered my services, and this book is the result. It is meant to be part historical adventure and part *Physician's Desk Reference,* explaining how garlic works and exactly what it can and cannot be used for.

In the process of sifting through the mountain of data I have acquired over two decades, I glanced through a number of books about garlic. The first thing that struck me as odd, was their lack of a true sense of this incredible herb's history. Most of them did mention the Greeks, Romans, and Egyptians, but only in passing. No one traced the origins of garlic back to the Sumerians of Abraham's time. But I did my homework and came up with an entire chapter on this fascinating period of herbal history.

Second, none of the garlic books published thus far have delved into any of the ancient herbals. Here was a real treasure trove of information about garlic's use in ancient times. Most of the other garlic books dredge up garlic's anti-Dracula actions in Transylvania, but I went back even further, to ancient Mesopotamia, where the lore about garlic warding off evil spirits began.

Third, I was always disappointed to find how general and limited in scope the data was on garlic's many wonderful benefits. While it is true that some authors did include more material on this than others, it still never seemed to be enough, especially when you consider the wealth of information that abounds in the medical and scientific literature on garlic's healing virtues. I wanted at least one major chapter on garlic's role in disease management, and as things turned out, this is the biggest section of the book. The health problems covered range from acne to worms and include not only self-help information but also plenty of literature citations to support the therapies listed.

After completing this comprehensive overview, I paused to reread what I had written. I felt that something was missing, but I hadn't a clue as to what it was. So I nibbled on some more garlic one night and put on my Gilroy Garlic Festival thinking cap, and lo and behold, those sulphur fumes cleared out the cobwebs from my mind. The book needed a chapter on medicinal preparations that use garlic, and what better place to locate this "garlic pharmacy" than right after the chapter on disease management.

Garlic is celebrated around the world in a growing number of annual festivals. I have attended a few myself (that's where I got my thinking cap) and describe them in Chapter Seven.

The final chapter is a recipe section for those wanting to fix foods flavored with a lot of garlic. But I didn't want recipes for the sake of recipes only. Instead, I wanted gourmet recipes with a sense of history about them—in other words, recipes with character. That's why I chose recipes from several different parts of the world to ensure ethnic diversity.

Finally, an appendix was attached with resources for obtaining additional information pertaining to garlic.

The result is a repair manual for your body involving the single greatest herbal tool which Nature has bequeathed to the human race—all-purpose, anytime, full-strength garlic! Let your fingers walk through these "yellow pages" of garlic often to keep you healthy. The best compliment you could ever pay me or my publisher is to refer to this volume so frequently that it becomes worn out with handling. After all, there's nothing an author likes more than to see a dog-eared, well-read copy of his work in someone else's library.

—JOHN HEINERMAN, PH.D.
Salt Lake City

THE
Healing Benefits
OF
GARLIC

CHAPTER ONE

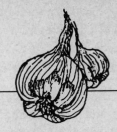

Out of Sumer: When Garlic was First Used

ENDURING DESERT AGONIES WITH GARLIC

THE archaeology of the ancient Near East has always been a muddled affair for scientists working there. Throughout the middle of the 19th to the 20th centuries, numerous excavations were made in various parts of Iraq to determine what the very earliest civilization may have been. Like the layers of an onion, hundreds of thousands of tons of sand were moved by hand in an enormous effort to uncover the remains of buildings buried for millennia.

The French, Germans, British, and Americans all dug in different places hoping to uncover magnificent treasures and more important artifacts, such as inscribed clay tablets called

4 THE HEALING BENEFITS OF GARLIC

cuneiform. As Erich Zehren has so vividly depicted in his classic work *The Crescent and the Bull: A Survey of Archaeology in the Near East* (New York: Hawthorn Books, Inc., 1961), they endured sheer hell for the sake of science:

> They worked in a nightmare environment of fleas, ticks and flies. During the day these persistent insects crept into their eyes, noses and ears. To take a breath meant getting them into one's windpipe, where they were swallowed with one's meals. They were dangerous, almost irresistible, carriers of disease.

A French vice-consul by the name of Ernest de Sarzec was one of those attracted to the Iraqi port city of Basra, which lies at the junction of the Euphrates and Tigris Rivers. Basra was the site of repeated conflicts between Iran and Iraq during the recent war between them. It was the site again of deadly engagements between Saddam Hussein's men and the troops involved in the Desert Storm operation to liberate Kuwait from Iraqi possession.

One morning Sarzec arose from his cot and absent-mindedly slipped into his shoes before first checking them out. A slumbering scorpion let him know in no uncertain terms exactly how it felt about having its sleep so rudely interrupted by a human foot. One of the Bedouin servants hired by Sarzec recommended an old desert remedy for the poor Frenchman's swollen, painful foot.

The servant peeled several cloves of garlic and crushed them on a flat stone with the butt of his riflestock. He then scooped up the crushed material into the palm of his open hand with the blade of his dagger and proceeded to drool some of his own saliva into his hand, at the same time stirring this curious mixture with his other forefinger. After garlic and spittle were thoroughly mixed together, he slapped the moist vegetable poultice directly onto the spot where Sarzec had been stung. Within minutes, the pain began to subside as the enzymatic action of the saliva in combination with sulphur components of the garlic made their way into the Frenchman's bloodstream, where they began to neutralize the deadly effects of this arachnid's venom.

On another occasion, while traveling a great distance to the north of Basra with some native guides in search of fabled ruins, he stopped to quench his thirst from a brackish pool of water that even the jackals avoided. He promptly took sick with a raging fever and frightful diarrhea.

Again his faithful Bedouin servant came to the rescue. This time the fellow made a fire and hung a coffee pot full of water over it on an iron tripod. When the water had sufficiently boiled, he put half a dozen peeled, chopped garlic cloves into the pot, put the lid back on, and let the brew simmer for 30 minutes. Several cupfuls of this garlic broth were then forced down Sarzec every couple of hours. Over the next 36 hours his condition improved so much that he was able to get up from his sick bed and proceed on his way.

LOCATING SUMER

Until Sarzec's historic discovery at the rubbish heaps of Telloh, the Sumerians and their city of Sumer had been considered mythical. Throughout the 19th century a succession of European linguists energetically denied that there had ever been such a people. Yet none of them could explain the rationale to the place name cited in Genesis 10:10, which describes the boundaries of the immense territory ruled by wicked King Nimrod of Tower of Babel fame: "And the beginning of his kingdom was Babel, and Erech, and Accad, and Calneh, *in the land of Shinar.*"

Some, like Sarzec, believed Shinar to be synonymous with Sumer and pressed forward in spite of all the odds and hardships against them in hopes of finding enough evidence to confirm the reality of Sumer. It was in the region of hills called Telloh that he found, after years of digging, a collection of more than 30,000 inscribed tablets, well arranged and larger than even those of the Nineveh library discovered by Hormuzd Rassam in 1854.

Rassam had been on the trail of Assurbanipal, the last great king of Assyria before its downfall. This particular king had assembled, from all the important cities of Mesopotamia, tens of thousands of clay tablets with mysterious cuneiform characters on them. They covered a wide range of subjects ranging from agriculture and domestic matters to religion and medicine. Among them were tablets devoted exclusively to botanical remedies. Rassam had all of the tablets carefully packed and shipped to London, where it took three decades to catalogue this great library. Eventually, the great Assyriologist R. Campbell Thompson translated the tablets dealing with medicinal agents into *The Assyrian Herbal.*

The vast collection discovered by Sarzec preceded Rassam's find by at least another one and a half millennia, and it proved the existence of a people called Sumerians. French archaeologists were ecstatic, as were scholars over the rest of Europe, in America, and throughout the world.

The French kept digging at Telloh until the middle 1930s, when they returned to Paris, rich with their experiences and treasures. By that time the learned world had ascertained that the Telloh mound concealed the ruins of a marvelous Sumerian city called Lagash.

Entire generations of its princes emerged from a shadowy past already at an end a thousand years before Moses was born and much more remote than the days of Abraham. Lagash, therefore, became an important source of archaeological information and remains so at the present time, over a century after its discovery.

When Garlic was First Used

It was here in Sumeria somewhere around 2300 B.C. that garlic first came into prominence. When the area first became inhabited, scholars believe it was an unhealthy collection of bogs and marshes requiring the construction of an extensive and elaborate drainage system to make living conditions tolerable. Zehren's description of present environment is considered a good reflection of its conditions four millennia ago:

> In the summer it is either waterlogged or quite arid and swept by hot sandstorms. It is only in the short winter that conditions are anything like tolerable for the European. Nature fights more obstinately there than in northern Mesopotamia to prevent the unearthing of human settlements buried in both areas for thousands of years. Fever and plague, swarms of gnats, snakes, hornets and scorpions, floods, sandstorms and humid or torrid heat assault the explorer.

Records from the princes of Lagash, as well as others brought to light later by Germans digging south of the ancient sites of Babylon and Nippur, indicate that garlic was extensively employed in Nimrod's time for the following conditions:

1. As an infusion for the reduction of fevers. Garlic, probably coarsely cut, was steeped in some

type of covered clay pot in boiling water for about half an hour.

2. As a decoction for loose bowels. In such cases, coarsely chopped garlic would be simmered in a covered clay pot over a medium fire. At some point (it was never specified just when) a few pieces of hardened myrrh gum were thrown into the pot, the lid put back on, and the mixture permitted to simmer some more.

3. As a fomentation for painful swellings. Either an infusion or decoction would be made up first. Then some type of cloth material would be dipped into the liquid solution, loosely wrung out, and applied over the affected area as hot as the patient could stand it without burning the skin. It is not known whether another dry cloth was put over this to retain the heat as long as possible.

4. As a liniment for strained muscles or pulled ligaments. Some unspecified kinds of animal grease were used to gently simmer garlic cloves and eucalyptus leaves. After the material had been allowed to cool and set up, it was rubbed on the body to eradicate stiffness and soreness.

5. As a tincture for intestinal parasites and a liniment substitute. Garlic was soaked in beer from one full moon to the next and regular swigs of it were guzzled down to get rid of worms or else rubbed on the skin for common aches and pains.

6. As a general tonic for feeling good. Made in much the same way that a tincture is today, garlic tonic was popular for improving the heart, strengthening digestion, and increasing personal bravery in soldiers.

BEER, BREAD & GARLIC, SUMERIAN STYLE

In 1992, one of my staff, Matthew Fountaine, and I traveled to Camp Verde, Arizona, where I was the opening and closing speaker at the Second Annual "Arizona's Own Garlic Festival." About 5,000 people attended the two-day event. Some of the exhibits featured garlic bread, of course, and (wouldn't you know it) garlic beer. The fellow serving up the suds claimed to have invented the world's *first* garlic beer. I didn't have the heart to inform him that he was 4,000 years too late.

According to some of the ancient texts described earlier, beer was a Sumerian invention. From all that historians can determine, beer played an important part in Sumerian society and was consumed by men and women from all social classes. In the Sumerian and Akkadian dictionaries currently being compiled by scholars, the word for beer crops up in contexts relating to medicine, ritual, and myth. Parlors serving plain beer, rose- or frankinscence-scented beer, honey-sweetened beer, and garlic beer received special mention in the laws codified by Hammurabi in the 18th century B.C. Stiff penalties were levied on proprietors who overcharged customers (death by drowning) or who failed to notify authorities of the presence of criminals in their establishments (execution). High priestesses who were caught in such ancient pubs were condemned to death by burning.

In combing the Sumerian literature recently, Solomon Katz, a bioanthropologist at The University Museum, University of Pennsylvania, and Fritz Maytag, president of Anchor Brewing Company of San Francisco, decided to examine the "Hymn of Ninkasi." This document, which dates to about 1800 B.C., sings the praises of the Sumerian goddess of brewing. The text, known from tablets found at Nippur, Sippar, and Larsa, had been translated by Miguel

Civil of the Oriental Institute of the University of Chicago in 1964. Coded within the hymn is an ancient recipe for beer. Katz and Maytag returned to the hymn over and over before attempting to brew this ancient recipe. On several occasions they met with Civil to discuss parts of the text that were vague or ambiguous. In responding to their questions, Civil was led to refine his translation of certain Sumerian words such as honey, wine and garlic. He made a new translation of the hymn, which allowed Katz and Maytag to recreate Sumerian beer for the very first time.

Along the way, they made an intriguing discovery. They found that the Sumerian use of barley coincided with both beer and bread. When the "Hymn to Ninkasi" was written, beer was made using bread. But *bappir*, the Sumerian bread, could be kept for long periods of time without spoiling, so it was a storable resource. They also noticed, from various annotations on *bappir* and beer in the Sumerian and Akkadian dictionaries now underway, that *bappir* was eaten only during food shortages. In essence, making bread was a convenient way to store the raw materials for brewing beer.

This raises an intriguing question: Did man once live by something other than mere bread alone? The English archaeologist/brewer James Death believed he did. In his book, *The Beer of the Bible* (London, 1877) he made a strong case for beer's primacy, stating, "I adduce reasons to show that the manufacture of beer was the earliest art of primitive man; an art exceeding in antiquity that of the potter or of the wine maker, *and certainly that of the baker.*"

For anyone seriously interested in the wealth of material dealing with Sumerian brewing procedures and beer styles, I recommend the pioneering work on the subject by Hrozny, *Das Getreide im alten Babylonien* (The Cereal Grains of Ancient Babylon) (Vienna, 1914), wherein more than 25 Sumerian brews are identified in detail.

It is unclear what extent garlic may have played in the double role of bread-making and beer-brewing, but this spice showed up in several different types of beers, which were consumed for upset stomach, diarrhea, gas, heartburn, and sluggish liver activity. It may be that some of these very early garlic beers were used by physicians to disinfect wounds and cuts suffered by soldiers in battle.

Certainly we know this much about the first uses of garlic in Sumeria. The herb had definite medical purposes in helping to fight inflammation, stop infection, eliminate parasites, and restore vitality to the system. It is probably safe to say from a historical perspective that the Sumerians, and later the Romans (from whom all Italians are descended), invented not only garlic beer but also the garlic bread that went with it!

It was up to the Egyptians, Greeks, and Romans, however, to more fully utilize this wonderful herb on a grand scale.

CHAPTER TWO

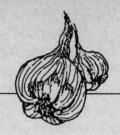

Pharoahs, Philosophers, and Gladiators: Only Their Breath Set Them Apart

WHEN EMPIRES AND GARLIC MET

MANY of the Old World kingdoms, which have either passed into oblivion or are but a shadow of their former greatness and glory, considered garlic to be one of the most important spices for feeding and healing the human body. Egyptians, Hebrews, Greeks, and Romans alike ate and drank and used this herb in many different ways.

The grand opus of ancient Egyptian medicine—a massive ten-volume work by H. Grapow entitled *Grundriss der Medizin der alten Ägypter* (Compendium of the Medicine of Ancient Egypt) 1954–1962—relates that one Hesy Re, Chief of Dentists and Physicians to the pyramid builders of the

Third Dynasty around 2600 B.C., plugged cavities with crushed garlic. At that time it wasn't in vogue to simply pull bad teeth out. In fact, just the opposite was the case— preserve them at all costs no matter how rotten to the roots they may have been. Re's method was to crush a peeled garlic clove in a stone mortar with a pestle and then smear some wild honey on the macerated pulp before inserting it directly on the royal toothache. The honey helped the garlic pulp stick to the cavity.

Some years ago while speaking at a National Health Federation convention in New Orleans, one of my own amalgam fillings fell out of a back molar. A throbbing pain soon ensued and I was hard-pressed to find a dentist over the weekend. So I went to a nearby grocery store and purchased several cloves of garlic and a small jar of peanut butter. Back in my hotel room, I peeled a garlic clove, pounded it flat with the bottom of a heavy glass ashtray, mixed it with a little peanut butter, and stuck it into the gaping hole. Within minutes the pain ceased and I managed very nicely for the rest of my stay. Upon returning home, my local dentist refilled it. Thus, because of something I had read in Grapow's colossal work years before, I was able to put to the test a 4500 year-old remedy with good success.

The Egyptians fed huge amounts of garlic to their Hebrew slaves in an effort to control the spread of epidemics that might arise from crowding so many people into small living quarters. And the Children of Israel themselves, from what the Bible and similar histories have to say, used garlic for flavoring their meals as well as for health reasons.

In the "Golden Age" of Greece, physicians and philosophers lived and worked side by side. Those like Hippocrates (460–380 B.C.) practiced the healing arts, while men such as Socrates, Plato, and Aristotle (circa 470–322 B.C.) debated the ethics of medicine as well other subjects of life in general. The doctor or *iatrós*, as he became known, was expert in diagnosing different symptoms and describing them with words that are an essential part of today's medical jargon: rheuma[tism], crisis, asthma, tetanos, anthrax, dysenteria, sepsis, ataxia, pleuritis, hypochondria, and so forth.

The oldest witness of Greek medicine is the epic poet Homer (850 B.C.). There are 147 wounds mentioned in his *Illiad* alone, suggesting that this was the main specialty treated by the *iatrós*. Crushed garlic, boiled garlic and wine-soaked garlic were often used in conjunction with other medicaments to prevent the onset of infection and to expedite the healing process.

It was Rome, the mightiest of the three civilizations dealt with in this chapter, that put garlic to some of its greatest and most diverse uses. Legion soldiers ate it with bread for strength; gladiators sometimes munched on whole cloves for endurance in the coliseums; some of the nobility drank a mixture of garlic and wine as an effective antidote against possible poisoning; physicians like Galen used it often during surgery as a disinfectant; and it was occasionally chopped and mixed in with the feed of domesticated animals to relieve intestinal gas due to foundering on new grass or too much grain.

This chapter is a short synopsis of some of these wonderful uses for one of the world's oldest medicinal and food herbs. Many of these discoveries have lain buried for decades in musty, old volumes of scholarly works dealing with each of these great empires. A walk back into time through these history books will enable us to see how cultures like our own in some respects came to rely upon a stinking herb with so many surprising virtues. For if anything set them apart from non-users, it would have been their unmistable garlic breath!

SULPHUR FOODS FOR PLAQUE CONTROL

Garlic and some other foods are rich in the mineral sulphur. The ancient Greek historian Herodotus wrote, "There is an inscription in Egyptian characters on the pyramid which records the quantity of radishes, onions, [and] garlic consumed by the laborers who constructed it; and I perfectly well remember that the interpreter who read the writing to me said that the money thus expended was 1600 talents of silver." In today's purchasing power, this is approximately 30 million U.S. dollars—a substantial investment!

Further evidence that these sulphur-bearing items occupied an important position in the Hebrew diet comes from one of the Five Books of Moses (Numbers 11:5) in the Old Testament. When the Children of Israel were with Moses in the wilderness and faced the prospect of going hungry for lack of adequate food, they complained, "We remember the fish, which we did eat in Egypt freely; the cucumbers, and the melons, and the leeks, and the onions, and the garlic; but now our soul is dried away: there is nothing at all, besides this manna, before our eyes."

One can easily discern just how health-giving the diet must have been for the Hebrews when they resided in Egypt. Certainly the fish gave them ample vitamin A and omega fatty acids, both of which do the heart good and bolster weak immune defenses. The cukes and melons would have been marvelous cleansing foods to purify the bloodstream and internal organs of toxins. And the radishes, onions, leeks, and garlic would have given the body different types of sulphur amino acids to help increase the production of white blood cells, killer T-cells, and macrophages—all vital parts of a strong immune system.

GARLIC IN THE TYPICAL HEBREW DIET

Garlic figured prominently in the preparation of various kinds of foods in the traditional Hebrew diet. One such item was the migratory insect called a locust. The head, wings, legs, and intestines were removed and only the flesh portion eaten. The usual method of preparation consisted of briefly soaking the insect in some garlic and onion juice before oven-roasting, sun-drying and salting it. Ancient rabbinical writings suggest that this "insect potato chip" was simply delicious!

Along with leeks and onions, garlic provided an aromatic quality to savory stews made with beans, lentils or peas. It was for one of these that Esau sold his birthright to Jacob in order to satisfy his gnawing hunger. The following recipe, with some modifications to accommodate modern taste preferences, is modeled after a stew similar to the one Jacob used to entice his brother.

OLD TESTAMENT STEW

1 cup dry lentils, rinsed
6 cups water
1 tsp. Worcestershire sauce
2 bay leaves
2 cloves garlic, minced
½ tsp. paprika
dash of ground cloves

¼ tsp. black pepper
2 cups carrots, quartered
4 medium potatoes, quartered
3 medium onions, quartered
1 tbsp. cornstarch
8 oz. ground lamb meat, browned

1. Cover lentils with water in a large pot. Bring to a boil and cook uncovered 30 minutes.

2. Add the vegetables, Worcestershire sauce, bay leaves, garlic, paprika, cloves, and black pepper. Cook, covered with a lid, for another 30 minutes.

3. Drain, reserving the broth. Set aside vegetables and lentils, then remove the bay leaves and discard.

4. Add enough water to reserved liquid, if necessary, to equal 2 cups. Return to the pot.

5. Whisk the cornstarch into ½ cup cool water until smooth, and slowly pour into the soup pot. Heat, stirring constantly until thickened.

6. Add previously browned lamb meat, lentils, and vegetables to soup pot. Heat and serve. Serves eight.

Reverend Cunningham Geikie's classic work, *The Life and Words of Christ* (London: Strahan & Co., Ltd., 1880), mentions a vegetable appetizer that graced many a Hebrew table in olden times. It consisted of endives, lettuce, and radishes which were dipped into a mixture of olive oil, chopped garlic, salt, and vinegar, and consumed with lipsmacking relish.

The evening meal was likely to end with one of a number of different fruits, such as dates, figs, melons, and pomegranates. In an era without refined sugar, the first two items were especially prized for their sweetness. During the much-celebrated Passover meal, a bowl of *charoseth* always accompanied the paschal lamb. As Dr. Geikie related, *charoseth* "was a dish which contained dates and figs and was a brick color, to remind them of the bricks and mortar of Egypt."

The manner in which this *charoseth* was consumed is interesting in and of itself. After a Jew had washed his hands again, he took two pieces of unleavened bread (part of the Passover meal), broke them in half, pronounced a blessing of thanksgiving, wrapped some bitter herbs dipped in the garlicky vinegar oil combination around a piece of broken bread, and then dipped it into the *charoseth*. After eating this symbolic food, another prayer of thanksgiving was rendered, followed by a chunk of the Passover lamb.

Having studied the Mediterannean diet for a number of years, and having observed the frequent use of garlic oil by many people in the Near East, I have noticed two definite health advantages for many of them. First of all, their serum triglycerides and cholesterol level are lower than those of many people in the West. Second, they have far less incidence of sugar diabetes than Europeans and North Americans do. Both can be directly attributed to the cholesterol-lowering and sugar-stabilizing properties of this marvelous spice.

GETTING RID OF THE DREADED 'UKHEDU'

The Egyptians used garlic for cleaning out their colons. Different ancient medical papyri contain numerous references to the anus. As one author put it, "They apparently took the anus as the center and stronghold of decay."

Worry about decay must have slowly grown to a national concern. It governed daily life even in the time of Herodotus (5th century B.C.): "For three consecutive days in every month they purge themselves, pursuing after health by means of emetics and drenches; for they think it is from the food they eat that all sicknesses come to men."

The most frightening aspects of feces to the average Egyptian was that they contained a pernicious thing called *ukhedu. Ukhedu* lay there dormant but might arise and settle anywhere in the body. The closest English definition for this complex Egyptian term is "rotten stuff par excellence" or just plain anal "rot." The discharge of gas from the rectum meant that *ukhedu* was fast at work and an Egyptian wasted no time in consulting a physician who specialized in giving enemas. Warm garlic enemas were the most preferable. These were made by boiling peeled and chopped garlic cloves in water, then cooling the "tea" to lukewarm before judiciously administering it through an ox horn into the rectum of the reclining patient. Garlic was the treatment of choice for many an Egyptian with fear in his mind and putrefaction in his colon.

This attention to the anus can be seen in a bit of history cited by author Jürgen Thorwald in his classic work, *Science and Secrets of Early Medicine* (New York: Harcourt, Brace & World, 1963). An inscription over the tomb of one of the court physicians uncovered in 1911 by archaeologists read in part, "Guardian of the Royal Bowel Movement"! We presume that this fellow kept food moving through the Pharoah's digestive tract while the latter concentrated on regulating the affairs of state. Undoubtedly, garlic played a significant role in all of this.

AN EGYPTIAN REMEDY FOR HYSTERIA

A remarkable medical prescription for hysteria from ancient Egypt appeared in Volume 3 of the *Annals of Medical History* (1921).

The specific remedy called for camphor, valerian, asafoetida and garlic to be soaked in strong wine, after which the liquid was to be strained and given in small amounts to hysterical patients.

The prescription works, as my own research has proven. More intriguing is the fact that it works better when the ingredients have had a chance to age or slightly ferment as opposed to using them fresh. The aging process seems to enhance this formula's success. In Asiatic countries such as China, Korea, and Japan, it has been a common practice to age meat, eggs, vegetables, and garlic by storing them in special containers or, as in the case of duck eggs, burying them for lengthy periods of time. Aging is said to improve their flavor and nutritional goodness.

PAIN-KILLING AGENTS IN HIPPOCRATIC MEDICINE

Around the year 400 B.C., Hippocrates would have been somewhere in his sixties and perhaps practicing in his home island of Cos. He had lived through the age of Pericles, the building of the Parthenon, the Great Plague of Athens, the fall of Athens to the Spartans, many a première of Sophocles, Euripides, and Aristophanes, and the last years of Socrates. In Plato's dialogues Socrates speaks of him with the utmost respect, and so does Aristotle. We can be sure that he really existed, but we do not know for sure what he really said, let alone discovered. The Hippocratic Collection

represents not his collected works but rather the remains of
a library, possibly that of his medical school at Cos. It is a
potpourri of about seventy anonymous essays and frag-
ments varying in length from one to a few pages and is very
uneven in value. A few essays contain passages worthy of
the master; others are poor, incomplete, or contradictory.
The voice of Hippocrates, which guided men for 2,200 years,
comes through somewhat blurred, as if it arose from the
bottom of a well. But let there be no misunderstanding: if
medicine was not born in ancient Greece, it was certainly
reborn there.

The Hippocratic Collection is at its best in matters surgical, and it has a lot to say about wounds. In those days,
Greek physicians spent much of their time traveling—or, to
use their own term, doing *epidemics*. The word has radically
changed its meaning, for it meant "visits to places"; several
Hippocratic books are titled *Epidemics*. However, the *iatrós*
or doctor also had a permanent working place in town called
the *iatréion*. This was a truly professional establishment,
roomy, with "two kinds of light, the ordinary and the artificial . . . either direct or oblique," and equipped with surgical
instruments, natural drugs, apparatus, and perhaps scrolls
of medical literature. The physician himself, though not
aseptic, was spotless, neat, and reassuring—even perfumed.

Two popular drugs were opium and garlic. Evidence
discovered in 1937 by Greek archaeologists suggests that
ripe poppy capsules were slit to extract their raw opium,
which was then compounded with expressed garlic juice and
added to wine. This mixture was given to patients requiring
surgery or suffering from wounds or inflammation to ease
their excruciating pain.

Bandages were also soaked in this drugged wine and
used to dress wounds; the opium-garlic mixture penetrated

through the skin and into the bloodstream, where it quickly acted as an efficient anodyne to soothe or relieve pain.

Greek medicine, while remarkable in some areas, was questionable in other matters. For instance, patients with white and "pure" pus were said to have a better prognosis than those with "bad" pus. If the pus stank, it was an ominous sign; but if it was odorless and flowed "pure and white," it was taken to be a good omen.

This medical error may explain why historians have never found a direct reference in any of the Hippocratic literature to the antibacterial properties of garlic; they never used it that way. The common *iatrós* of Hippocrates' time knew that garlic had a mysterious synergism with opium and could quickly kill pain in the suffering patient. He understood that if garlic was added to wine, an antiseptic wound wash would result. But he was always careful never to use too much garlic for fear of stopping the production of "pure" pus in his patient. Thus the infection continued unchecked. Little wonder, then, that the mortality rate for wounded patients was well over 60 percent. The old adage that the cure was a success but unfortunately the patient died may in fact have originated in ancient Greece.

THE MILITARY USE OF GARLIC IN ANCIENT ROME

Between the 4th and 3rd centuries B.C., a huge group of pagan people invaded and occupied much of Europe just north of the Alps. Called the Celts, they were in control of a vast area that stretched from Ireland and Spain in the west to parts of Eastern Europe. But in the latter part of the 3rd century B.C., a steady reversal of Celtic fortunes began with a number of major military engagements initiated by the Romans.

Historians of that time and later periods spoke of the mighty victories won by Roman legions in the Battle of Telamon in Italy (225 B.C.), at Gallia Cisalpina (Gaul on the Italian side of the Alps) in 191 B.C., and in southern Gaul in the 2nd century B.C. In the middle of the 1st century B.C., the Romans turned their attention to Gaul, which was finally subjugated by Julius Caesar in 50 B.C., and, under the emperors Augustus and Tiberius, the remainder of Celtic Europe was subdued. By 84 A.D., the armies of the Roman governor Agricola reached northern Scotland, marking the end of most of the Celtic world. Only Ireland remained untouched by the presence of Rome.

Roman generals depended upon a small selection of particular foods to provide their weary foot soldiers with the necessary strength to march incredible distances over rough and unfriendly terrain in the worst kinds of weather imaginable. Such food had to be easy to carry and prepare, yet able to meet the energy requirements of exhausted troops expected to tramp for hundreds of miles and fight like tigers in fierce battles.

When perusing the old medical and scientific literature of that period from men like Pliny the Elder (he wrote his massive 37-volume *Historia naturalis* between 75–77 A.D.), Cornelius Celsus (he wrote his 3-volume work, *De medicina* between 30–40 A.D.), and Claudius Galen (his 22-volume medical encyclopedia was written in Greek and translated into Latin in the 2nd Century A.D.), one discovers that garlic was frequently used along with many different food staples.

Roman army rations fell into three main forms: solid food, slops or gruel, and nourishing drinks. Wild game caught, killed, and cooked along the way would be made into a stew containing ripe pomegranate juice, crushed and salted pistachio nuts, and chopped garlic clove. (The pomegranates, pistachios, and garlic were transported with each legion expedition.) Meals like this were fixed when the men had time to stop, rest, and do some hunting.

More often than not, slops or gruels were the mainstay, especially when commanders had their forces on the move. Three favorite gruels were the following: (1) boiled millet with white wine; (2) boiled barley diluted with white wine; and (3) boiled barley, honey, pomegranate and garlic. It seems that gruel #3 was for medicinal as well as chow purposes, probably to keep the soldiers' guts free of intestinal parasites as they crossed strange lands and drank unsanitary water.

It also appears that legumes such as lentils and chickpeas were occasionally eaten by some of these legions, especially when they were garrisoned in one spot for a long time. Here again garlic as well as leek, onion, and salt came into play, giving these legume dishes a little flavor.

Undoubtedly, though, it was a variety of nourishing drinks that gave the Roman military their greatest bursts of energy and helped them to endure rougher conditions than even today's U.S. Army troops had to put up with in the recent "Desert Storm" operations in the Mideast. One drink simply consisted of honey and the fermented juice of white grapes. This is the same wine vinegar that was offered to the crucified Christ at Calvary by a Roman soldier.

Two other drinks contained slightly aged garlic. The ingredients, including crushed garlic, were fermented in flagons before being put into leather skins or canteens, which the soldiers carried on their expeditions. This aging process seems to have kept enzyme activity and some of the B-complex vitamin group (thiamine, riboflavin, biotin, choline, folic acid, niacin, and pangamic acid) intact.

The first of these consisted of cooked barley, crushed garlic, and white wine. The other included the same boiled barley and its water with crushed garlic, mashed ripe pomegranate, and dark honey. Having experimented with a few of these myself, I can attest to their remarkable ability to produce greater physical endurance when no other forms of nourishment are available.

GALEN AND THE GLADIATORS

Rome's greatest physician was Claudius Galen, considered the father of modern pathology. Born in 130 A.D. in Pergamon, on the coast of Asia Minor, he spent 24 of his adult years in Rome, where he rose to the position of court physician to Marcus Aurelius. He had no brothers or sisters, was never married, left no pupils, and doesn't mention any close friends. His one and only idol was Hippocrates. The Hippocratic Collection had already gathered five hundred years of dust when he revived it, adopted it as if he were its new messiah (which he surely was) and wrote much about it that is extremely valuable to us today. Indeed, his comments on the Hippocratic books are usually longer than the books themselves.

Yet while his medicine was essentially Hippocratic, Galen had been to the Alexandrian school. For all his faults, his scientific horizon reached at least one order of magnitude beyond that of Hippocrates: he practiced dissection and experiment.

Pergamon was a Greek city and had nothing to do with gladiators, but when the Romans came, the conquerors could not do without their favorite show. On Greek soil, however, the first reaction was horror, and some Greek cities went as far as forbidding gladiatorial games altogether. The Romans solved the problem by a technique of immunization: they organized combats anyway, but stopped them, at first, as soon as blood appeared. Gradually, the public became accustomed to gore and expected it. By the time Galen was 28 years old, Pergamon had full gladiatorial games and needed a surgeon. This is what Galen wrote about his appointment:

> On my return from Alexandria to my native land, while still a young man in my 28th year, I had the good fortune to work out a successful dressing for wounded nerves and tendons. I demonstrated this to physician friends not only in Pergamon, but in neighboring cities so that they might confirm my findings by experiment. The treatment coming, I know now how, to the knowledge of the Pontifex of our city [president of the games], he entrusted me with the care of the gladiators while still a young man, for I was arriving at my 29th year . . .
>
> Since many died in previous years [and] not one of those treated by me died, the succeeding Pontifex appointed me likewise.

Galen's "successful dressing" is more precisely a sauce. It could have been an improvement over local practice, but surely not over the Hippocratic school of medicine:

> Though previous gladiatorial physicians bathed the wound in hot water and put on a dressing of wheat flour moderately cooked in a mixture of oil and water, I omitted the water entirely and made the dressing of flour and chopped garlic in oil and poured an additional small amount of oil over it. The result was excellent, for not one of my cases died, though fatalities were numerous previously.

He also employed wine, the trustiest friend of all wounded Greeks:

> As I have previously explained, it is necessary to keep the wound continually moist, because if the dress-

ings dry out, the ulcer becomes inflamed. This is true especially in summer, at which time when the pontifices of Pergamon were celebrating the appointed gladitorial games. I cured the most seriously injured by covering the wounds by a cloth wet with astringent garlic wine kept moist both day and night by a superimposed sponge.

Whereas the Greek *iatrós* had been hesitant to use too much garlic for fear of killing off the "pure" pus, Galen's pathological training convinced him that there was no such thing as "good" pus—that, in fact, it was all bad. Therefore, he employed garlic and similar antibiotics extensively in his medical practice. His favorite uses for it were in the forms of a liquid salve or a vinegary wine. Either way, the garlic was capable of killing harmful bacteria, thereby preventing the onset of further infection.

His choice of garlic made sense for another reason: when combined with other herbs, it helped to stop bleeding. Galen relied heavily on locally applied "styptics." The best of his mixtures, he said, was made as follows: garlic, one part; frankincense, one part; aloes, one part; mix with egg white to the consistency of honey; and add a pinch of clippings from the fur of a wild March hare. He used it "perfectly safely" on a wound exposing the membranous coverings of the brain and spinal cord (known as the meninges) of one gladiator.

As laudable and heroic as his efforts were in staunching the bleeding of many injured fighters, Galen never learned how to apply a simple tourniquet. His first aid in case of hemorrhage was to raise the injured part, put a finger into the wound, find the gaping vessels, and compress them "gently, without causing pain." If this didn't stop the bleeding, then have "an assistant who co-operates with you, and in the manner described compresses for you the places in which you are in need of it."

If both of these failed, then came the herbal styptic mixture described above. A modified version called for only "garlic, one part; myrrh, one part; mix with honey and apply." The gladiators whom he treated were undoubtedly grateful that he knew something about herbs and finger compression, if not about tourniquets!

AN ANTIDOTE FOR POISONING

An even more amazing but somewhat bizarre use for garlic came about during the reign of the Emperor Claudius in mid-October, 54 A.D. It happened quite by accident and was probably never intended to be an effective antidote. But for a very brief period of time—no more than several hours at the most—it saved one man's life.

When Nero's mother, Agrippina, married the Emperor Claudius, she persuaded him to adopt her son. Her next order of business was to poison her husband so that Nero could inherit the throne. An undisclosed poison was infused into a fine and delicious mushroom of a kind of which Claudius was known to be particularly fond, and his murderous wife saw to it that he received this special mushroom by serving it to him with her own hand.

After tasting it he became very quiet and then called for the rest of his meal and some wine. Unfortunately for Agrippina and her fellow plotters, he ate several dishes that were heavily seasoned with garlic. He was carried off to his bed chambers quite senseless, but as the historians inform us, all of that garlic and wine apparently weakened the effects of the poison.

Since we don't know what specific poison was used, we can only conjecture at this point that the combination of fermented wine and the strong sulphur amino acids from the garlic somehow neutralized enough of the ingested toxin within Claudius' liver to keep it from doing greater damage.

I recall an interesting episode in which a friend of mine was spared the deadly effects of ptomaine poisoning. "My other three business partners got sicker than dogs," he remembered, "but I barely noticed any effects from the apparently spoiled meat we had consumed." I asked what he had eaten that might have varied from what his partners ate. "I had a large Caesar salad and several helpings of garlic bread while waiting for the rest of my meal," he replied. That and the dark Bavarian beer he drank probably worked for him just as the garlic and wine had done for Claudius.

To conclude our palace intrigue narrative, Agrippina instructed "the faithless physician" beside her to "tickle the throat of the sufferer with a poisoned feather." Before the morning of October 13th, 54 A.D., Claudius was dead and Nero finally ascended the throne.

Truly, garlic has seen some interesting and unusual applications within the course of human history.

CHAPTER THREE

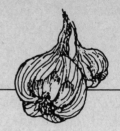

Garlic Lore from the Ancient Herbals

WARDING OFF DEVILS & DISEASES

VAMPIRES, those terrifying creatures that rise from the dead and suck the blood of sleeping humans, have thrilled and terrified people since ancient times. British novelist Bram Stoker moved the vampire from Slavic legend to popular culture when he published *Dracula* in 1897, for the Transylvanian vampire count was an instant sensation. Beginning with Bela Lugosi's classic portrayal in 1931, over a dozen Dracula movies have kept the vampire legend alive. As a result, almost everyone knows that garlic is a tried and true vampire repellent.

The notion that garlic can be used to ward off evil is

thought to have originated in Transylvania sometime in the
16th century. However, the idea was already established in
the time of Noah, when the world's first known herbal was
introduced to mankind.

One of the Dead Sea Scrolls, the "Book of Jubilees,"
written in 100 B.C., informs us of the following (10:7–14):

> And the Lord our God spoke to us [his angels] so
> that we might bind all of them [the evil spirits] . . .
>
> And he told one of us to teach Noah all of their
> healing . . . And we acted in accord with all of his words
> . . . And the healing of their [evil spirits'] illnesses to-
> gether with their seductions we told Noah so that he
> might heal by means of herbs of the earth.
>
> And Noah wrote everything in a book just as we
> taught him according to every kind of healing. And the
> evil spirits were restrained from following the sons of
> Noah. And he gave everything which he wrote to Shem,
> his oldest son, because he loved him much more than
> all of his sons.

Here two things become apparent. The first, of course,
is an implied connection between demons and disease—that
the former induces the latter. Second, we find reference to
the very first botanical records.

A Chaldean historian named Berosus, who lived between 500 and 400 B.C. and whom later historians such as
Flavius Josephus often quoted, claimed that the best herbs
to drive demons away were such foul-smelling ones as garlic, onion, fleabane, wormwood, and the like.

As scholar R. Campbell Thompson has shown from his
own translations of original cuneiform texts, the use of garlic
for keeping away evil influences was in full swing in ancient
Mesopotamia. His two-volume work, *The Devils and Evil
Spirits of Babylonia* (London: Luzac & Co., 1903) readily bears
this out.

A branch of tamarisk or clove of garlic were held aloft in the hand during the exorcism which was to repel the attacks of demons and lay them under a ban, and this shows that they were possessed of magical power. . . . This use of branches in magic shows that the early inhabitants of Babylonia were in no wise different from other nations in believing that trees were inhabited by spirits or gods [and could be used for protection against evil].

Thompson, a renowned Assyriologist, discovered in his translation of such clay tablets that the early inhabitants of Mesopotamia often hung garlic and other noxious herbs about their places to keep invisible and unwanted hosts away. "In order to prevent the entrance of demons into the house the Assyrians hung up various plants near the door," he wrote, and they followed with this invocation: "The flea-bane on the lintel of the door I have hung, St. Johnswort, garlic, and wheatears on the latch I have hung, with a halter as a roving ass thy body I restrain."

Many other Old World cultures in ancient times believed that garlic and onion held special virtues for warding off devil-induced sicknesses and that the gods had inspired men to eat of these herbs and use them in their homes. Consider the Israelites in Egypt. Shortly before the Lord smote all of the firstborn with a terrible plague of death, He instructed his servant Moses to have the Israelites sprinkle lamb's blood on the outside of their doorways and then to consume the roasted meat with "bitter herbs." This afforded them the protection they needed. It is said on good authority that two of those herbs were garlic and onion.

In modern times such thinking seems antiquated, if not foolish. Medical science has established that contagious diseases are spread by harmful bacteria or viruses. As will be shown in a later chapter, the strong sulphur amino acids emitted from garlic are decidedly antibacterial and antiviral in nature. Their presence disinfects the air, the body, and whatever else their overpowering odors come into contact with. This helps explain how garlic worked anciently as an effective natural antibiotic, though its effects were misinterpreted as having demons keep their distance.

An Assyrian Herbal

One of the many research monographs written by Dr. Thompson but never widely circulated or published in regular book form was *The Assyrian Herbal.* I am indebted to my colleague Alfred Bush, Curator of Special Collections at Princeton University, for providing me with a photocopy of this large and important work.

From it we can learn a few things about garlic or *sûmu*, as it came to be known in the Assyrian language. *Sûmu* was often boiled in milk and administered for "sick eyes" and "against grey hairs." Whether applied as an eyewash or scalp rinse or consumed internally was never indicated.

A piece of *sûmu* clove, however, was chewed periodically to help "fumigate" the mouth in order to get rid of "bad air." At first glance this might seem like a strange remedy for halitosis or bad breath. But upon closer examination, it referred more to evil influences entering such orifices of the body to work their mischief.

I once had a chance to test this practice against a pernicious influenza virus. During a month-long sojourn in the Soviet Union in the summer of 1979, I sat on a very long train ride next to some Russians who had the flu and who kept up a regular routine of coughing, hacking, sneezing, and blowing their noses.

My uneasiness grew because of the germs I knew were filling the air. I resolved to chew on some garlic cloves I had in my coat pocket. Although the odor annoyed my own senses for awhile, it afforded a protection I was glad of. Suffice it to say, whatever germs I might have inhaled didn't survive very long within my system, proving that the Assyrians were right in their recommendations.

Another condition for which they put garlic to full use, wrote Dr. Thompson, was in cases of dyspnea. This is simply shortness of breath, usually occurring during intense physical exertion or at high altitude, but which is also associated with heart disease or pulmonary disorders. A special type of drink was made, but no directions are given for its method of preparation or consumption.

Sûmu was regarded as an ideal treatment for getting rid of intestinal worms, encouraging proper kidney and bladder function, and alleviating diarrhea due to contaminated food or water. The juice was usually expressed from a number of raw cloves, mixed with a little wine, and then drunk straight.

THE HERBAL WISDOM OF KING SOLOMON

The great historian Flavius Josephus wrote his famous *Antiquities of the Jews* (Philadelphia: David McKay. William Whiston, translator) between 70 and 80 A.D. In Book Seven, Chapter Two, he wrote about "the sagacity and wisdom which God had bestowed upon Solomon" as being "so great, that he exceeded the ancient" in knowledge about many things.

Solomon wrote several books, one of which described "the virtues and properties of divers roots and herbs." In cases of exorcising demonic influences from those possessed of madness, he was said to be very skilled. Two of the herbs he used the most were valerian root and garlic clove. A small portion of either was inserted into the top of a large ring worn on one of his fingers. This was placed directly beneath the nostrils of the afflicted party, and the resulting fumes "drew out the demon."

Hard research is wanting to prove the efficacy of garlic or valerian in treating insanity. We know a little more about the latter in terms of calming anxiety and fear due to the presence of strong sedative components called valepotriates. It could be that the aromatic sulphur compounds in the former acted in much the same way that smelling salts or ammonia do in bringing someone out of a temporary mental stupor.

Another remarkable use for garlic was in the treatment of symptoms similar to an epileptic seizure but which were attributed to evil spirits. King Solomon wrote in his book of herbal wisdom that "the leek, the onion, or the garlic are all potent" against such influences. He recommended placing a small portion of any of these directly under the sufferer's nostrils or upon his forehead in hopes of driving the unseen malefactor away for good.

Also, the juice of any of these could be squeezed out and given orally, undiluted. Solomon claimed that if the possessed individual breathed or swallowed enough of their aroma or juice, an instant chain reaction would set up within the body. This agitation would compel the mischievous spirit within to depart from that particular tabernacle and seek someone else in which to take up residence.

Today, of course, the problem of epilepsy is controlled with prescription medications. It is doubtful that any members of the allium family would be able to compete with modern drugs in this arena. But in Solomon's time, it was part of the lore which may have worked for some.

THE WORLD'S MOST INFLUENTIAL HERBAL

Famous as the name of Hippocrates and the significance of the Hippocratic literature are, their direct influence upon the development of Western medicine and pharmacy was small compared with the deep and lasting effect of the teachings of Dioscorides, which flourished in the early part of the 1st century. Born in the village of Anazarba (not far from Tarsus, where Paul the Apostle grew up), Pedanios Dioscorides accompanied the army of Nero.

A close friend of his, a Roman army doctor by the name of Areius, suggested that he bring together into one volume all of the healing information about various botanicals and their properties which he had acquired in his many travels with Roman legions to different parts of the world. Thus was born *De materia medica libri quinque* (The Subject of Medicine in Five Volumes), which became the basis for European medicine for many, many centuries until modern times.

Whether Dioscorides actually practiced medicine remains uncertain, but he was with the Roman armies as they marched through Asia Minor, and his travels in Italy, Greece, Gaul, and Spain gave him extensive experience in the medical arts.

He not only described the plant, animal, and mineral drugs of his time and explained their effect but arranged his descriptions systematically, making him the first teacher of medicine and his treatise the most valuable and most used source in this field. The attempts of many later authors, up to the 17th century, to identify herbs in their native countries

according to descriptions given by Dioscorides for Mediterranean plants have caused many mistakes. They are, however, the best proof for the high authority accorded
Dioscorides.

De materia medica was translated into English in 1655
but not actually published until 1934. The contents of Dioscorides' five books, which were incorporated into a single
volume, were arranged as follows: Book I: Aromatics, oils,
ointments, trees; Book II: Living creatures, milk and dairy
products, cereals, and sharp herbs; Book III: Roots, juices,
herbs; Book IV: Herbs and roots; Book V: Vines and wines,
metallic ores.

This man knew the formation of leadplaster from fats
and lead oxide. He mentions the preparation of purified
woolfat and describes the making of extracts by maceration
followed by evaporation. He understood the process of ex-
pressing the fresh juice of plants and concentrating it by
exposure to the sun. He knew the difference between various gums, such as acacia, the gums of cherry, plum and
almond, and tragacanth. He explained the usual adultera-
tions and suggested means for discovering them. His re-
marks on the collection of drugs are excellent. His directions
for their storage were the first known and formed the basis
for many later ones.

AN ANTIDOTE FOR BITES

This most celebrated herbal of antiquity mentions
garlic often, but usually in connection with bites. To those
of us in the latter part of the 20th century, most bites are
nothing to worry about. We are unable to appreciate the
genuine concern and fear bites generated in ancient times.

There was even a medical *Book of Bites* which physicians in Egypt once consulted. The herbal of Dioscorides mentions bites a total of 329 times.

Garlic and related members of the allium family are spoken of more in relation to bites and poisons (another real fear then) than anything else. Dioscorides considered garlic to be one of the ultimate weapons in nature's vast arsenal for disarming the poisons resulting from bites, be they induced by man, animal, insect, or reptile.

One of his best remedies for neutralizing bite toxins called for equal amounts of cucumbers (crushed and unpeeled, garlic cloves (peeled and crushed), peppercorns (crushed), pomegranate juice, a few rust scrapings from any weathered sword blade or dagger, a little vinegar, and some small handfuls of coarse wheat flour and powdered myrrh gum. Everything was mixed together in a stone mortar with a pestle and then the pasty poultice was applied directly over the bite and left overnight. This helped to draw out whatever surface infection may have commenced.

At the same time, another formula was put together for the bite victim to take internally. This consisted of some garlic cloves (peeled and crushed) and squeezed juices from pomegranate and sour citrus fruits combined in a flask of wine, permitted to set overnight, and then given to the patient when the poultice was applied. Obviously this remedy had to be made up in advance and ready for immediate use whenever a bite of some type occurred.

REMARKABLE CURE FOR BURNS

One of the lesser known functions for which Dioscorides recommended garlic was in the treatment of simple burns. Yet this suggestion probably ranks as one of the more important treatments mentioned in his *De materia medica*. He felt that all of the alliums, particularly garlic and onion, held within them the power to restore growth to skin tissue which had been injured or damaged by fire.

Whether it is the sulphur amino acids present in these vegetable herbs that accomplishes such a feat remains a mystery. But this much is certain from the writings of Dioscorides—whenever expressed garlic or onion juice is mixed together with wild or raw honey (never heated) and applied directly to a burn as a dressing that is changed every day, over a matter of weeks tissue regeneration becomes quite evident.

It may be worth mentioning that two other doctors many centuries after Dioscorides copied his formula. The first of these was a French physician, Ambroise Paré (1510–1590).

With the increasing use of firearms, burns occurred frequently in the days of Paré, and surgeons were obviously anxious to improve their treatments. The traditional therapy consisted of cooling ointments, but some surgeons had more specific remedies. Paré had read from different herbals of his time, which quoted liberally from Dioscorides, about the use of garlic or onion juice and honey for treating burns. The few times he had employed just garlic and honey, he discovered to his own amazement what Dioscorides had known 1500 years before.

But Paré had never employed onion. In Piedmont in 1537, Paré, a young surgeon of 27 years, was attached to the army of the Marshal de Montejan in the third war between Francis I and Charles V. He relates his unique experience of combining garlic and onion together for the first time to treat a very serious third-degree burn, without either juicing

them or using honey. His narrative in the quaint English of
that period follows:

> One of the Marshall of *Montejan* his Kitchin boyes,
> fell by chance into a Caldron of Oyle being even almost
> boyling hot; I being called to dresse him, went to the
> next Apothecaries ... : there was present by chance a
> certaine old countrey woman, who hearing that I desired
> some Garlicke and Hony for a burne, perswaded mee at
> the first dressing, that I should insteade lay to raw On-
> ions and Garlicke beaten with a little salt; for so I should
> hinder the breaking out of blisters or pustules, as shee
> had found by certaine and frequent experience. Where-
> fore I thought good to try the force of her improved
> Medicine upon this greasy scullion. I the next day found
> those places of his body whereto the Garlicke and On-
> ions lay, to bee free from blisters, but the other parts
> which they had not touched, to be all blistered.

This account was taken from *The Workes of that famous
Chirurgion Ambroise Parey* (translated from Latin and compared with the French by Th. Johnson, London, 1634). The
result of this improved remedy given to him by an illiterate
peasant woman over the more tried and tested one proposed
by Dioscorides inspired Paré to try it again. Soon he had an
opportunity to do just that:

> It fell out a while after, that a German of *Montejan*
> his guard had his flasque full of Gunpouder set on fire,
> whereby his hands and face were grievously burnt: I
> being called, laid the Garlicke and Onions beaten as I
> formerly told you [with salt], to one half of his face, and
> to the other half I laid only Garlicke and Hony. At the
> second dressing I observed the part dressed with the
> Garlicke and Onions more free from blisters and excoria-
> tion, the other being stille troubled with some of both;
> whereby I gave credit to the newe Medicine.

The second individual to tap back into the ancient herbal lore of Dioscorides within modern times is a mainland Chinese medical doctor by the name of Xu Rongxiang. His new burn medication has attracted the attention of Western doctors everywhere. Rather than a transplantation technique or a genetically engineered tissue or hormone, it's an herbal salve that can be applied with a popsicle stick.

"In the past doctors have treated the complications of burns instead of curing the burned tissue," Dr. Xu told reporters. "But we went back to some ancient herbals, one in Greek [Dioscorides] and two in Chinese, to find those herbs which helped the body to repair injured skin." When pressed for details, he was reluctant to reveal the salve's specific ingredients until an international patent on his Moist Burn Ointment could be secured, but he did hint that it contained garlic, onion, sesame seeds, honey, salt, and other substances. He added that it fights infection by restoring oils and nutrients to damaged tissue. "We use nutrition, not drugs, to save lives," he said.

The results have been nothing short of amazing. Photographs document the progress of patients who have come to him with deep second-degree and superficial third-degree burns covering up to 94 percent of their bodies. Within months the same patients appear not only healed but virtually unscarred. Surgical grafts are still used where skin has been completely destroyed, but for the vast majority of burn injuries, Xu claims, his herbal ointment, borrowed in part from Dioscorides and Chinese herbalists of the past, is all that is needed—no bandages, no topical antibiotics, and no sterile isolation.

Now 34, Xu heads both his own institute and the Chinese government's national burn treatment center in Beijing. Fifty-five thousand Chinese patients have been successfully

treated with this miraculous therapy, according to information obtained from the Ministry of Public Health in
early 1992.

TEUTONIC HEADACHE RELIEF FROM 1000 A.D.

From an old and curious work of the 11th century
comes a surprisingly effective garlic remedy for getting rid
of migraines. Called the "Lacnunga" by scholars, this text
was an interesting amalgamation of Teutonic paganism,
Irish Christianity, and rehashed Greek medicine.

The original prescription was very complex and called
for 36 different plant ingredients, not to mention various
Latin chants to be sung at the time the formula was taken.
In attempting to re-create it, considerable time was involved
in separating the major herbs from the lesser ingredients.
After a good deal of trial and error, I narrowed them down
to radish, feverfew, betony, couchgrass, wormwood, hops,
yarrow, willow twigs, oak bark, and garlic.

My instincts suggested that this blend would make an
awful tasting tea, and they were correct. I substituted spring
water for the prescribed "holy water" because I couldn't
find a priest with the time or patience to come and bless the
water I intended making an herbal brew out of.

I used half teaspoons of every ingredient except the garlic; here I used two peeled and minced cloves. The coarser,
tougher botanicals were first simmered in a quart of water,
covered, for three minutes on low heat. Then the garlic was
added and simmered for an additional three minutes. Finally, the more delicate leafy or flowery ingredients (feverfew, betony, wormwood, and yarrow) were added, and the
pot was covered and removed from the heat to steep for
about forty minutes.

The solution was strained and one cup given warm to one of my female anthropology students who periodically suffered from migraines. While complaining of its repulsive, gagging taste, she nevertheless braved the bitterness and downed it with courage. Within about ten minutes her countenance improved considerably and she exclaimed, "I believe my headache is gone!"

I tried different ways to sweeten the brew, but without much success. Not only did some of the bitterness prevail, but every time a natural sweetener of some kind was added it diminished the medical effectiveness of the formula. The closest I ever came to making it half way palatable without affecting its action was to add a little pure vanilla to the finished product.

I also discovered in the course of my experiments that if a hand towel was soaked in some hot tea, wrung out, and then applied to the forehead and back of the neck, it would relieve even the worst headache within minutes. A second dry towel should be placed over the wet one to retain the heat as long as possible.

This may not be the most convenient or pleasant way to get rid of a migraine, but it is sure to work, nevertheless!

ASTHMA FORMULA GIVEN IN VISION

In an age when men dominated the religious and secular institutions of Europe, one woman achieved enough recognition to be considered almost an equal by many of them. Her name was Hildegarde of Bingen. Born in 1099 in the little German town of Böckelheim on the River Nahe, near Mainz, she was the daughter of a knight. For some unexplained reason—perhaps for economy, protection, or

development of special talents—she was placed in the Bene-
dictine convent at Disibodenberg at the age of eight. There
she was under the care of the Abbess Jutta, who saw to her
education. Hildegarde became her successor as head Abbess
in 1136 A.D.

From early childhood, this woman enjoyed the gift of
visions that became even more frequent, intense, and vivid
as she attained adulthood. She kept her extrasensory powers
to herself until she reached the age of 42, when she began
to write about them. Once her visions became known
throughout the religious community, they generated great
interest. Even someone as important as St. Bernard of
Clairvaux, who met her at Bingen while preaching the Second
Crusade, became convinced that she was a true prophetess
of the Lord. Recommendation from that quarter led to further recognition by the dignitaries of the Church, including
Pope Eugenius III himself.

About a dozen works are credited to her authorship,
her most important being the *Physica*, which discussed
plants and trees in relation to their medicinal properties. It
is the earliest work on natural history written in Germany,
and is, therefore, considered the foundation of botanical
study. Later 16th century works by Brunfels, Fuchs, and
Bock—the so called "German fathers of modern botany"—
were directly influenced by Hildegarde's volume.

A number of her visions have been preserved on rolls
of parchment, which have turned yellow with time, but they
can still be admired and studied by scholars in the European
museums that own them.

In one of these scrolls, she relates how an angel showed
her that the disease of the lungs which men called asthma
could be remedied with two simple herbs, hyssop and garlic.
The angel instructed her to make a plain broth from a handful of green hyssop tops and two garlic cloves. These were

to be cleaned, coarsely chopped, added to a pot of water, and cooked over a slow fire until ready to use.

For coughing or spitting up blood, the angel showed her how the addition of all-heal or woundwort to the same broth would dramatically reverse such hemorrhaging within minutes after being consumed. As for consumption, or what we now term tuberculosis, her heavenly visitor suggested adding lavender blossoms and comfrey leaf to the above hyssop-garlic broth.

It appears that the hyssop-garlic combination was an important remedy base to work from in treating various kinds of pulmonary disorders.

GARLIC AS YOU NEVER KNEW IT

One of the most singular treatises I came across while pursuing the study of garlic in damp and drafty European libraries and museums was *An Old Icelandic Medical Miscellany*. It was discovered by a scholar in Dublin who was cataloguing Celtic manuscripts. A portion of it is dated to the late 15th century, while other sections have been traced to the 13th and 14th centuries.

A chap named Henning Larsen translated it into English, and the work was subsequently published in a very limited edition. The portion covering garlic is found on pages 56 and 142–43 and is reproduced here for the first time:

> Allium is garlic. It is hot and dry in the fourth degree. If one eats it or rubs himself with it, that helps for the sting of vipers and of intestinal worms. And all harmful snakes flee before its smell. If it is boiled with oil, that makes a good ointment for all poisonous bites

and for broken bones and for a swelling or pain in the
bladder. If one boils garlic with honey and drinks, this
is good for lung disease; and so also if it is eaten with
vinegar. If a man eats it with centaury grass, it is good
for dropsy [edema]. Garlic drunk with wine gives a ca-
tharsis [bowel evacuation], and is good for jaundice [of
the liver]. If one boils it with beans and rubs his temples
with it, that is good for headache. But if it is crushed
with goose-fat and put in the ears, that helps for earache. If it is boiled, it is good for cough and drives away
illness and makes the voice bright. If one boils garlic in
porridge and eats, that is good for tenesmus [painful
straining of the bladder or bowels]. If it is crushed with
paunch-fat of swine it is good to apply to a swelling. If
one eats garlic while fasting, strange waters will not
harm him when he comes into strange places.

"FOUR THIEVES' VINEGAR"

Probably the single greatest garlic invention of the
Middle Ages was a remarkable formula devised by four
criminals. Called "Four Thieves' Vinegar" after the nature
of their crimes, it prevented them from getting sick as they
ravaged the bodies of unlucky victims of the bubonic
plague, which swept over many countries claiming millions
in its wake.

Thousands of Crusaders returning home from their so-
journs in the Holy Land brought with them this notorious
epidemic. Its appearance in the mid-14th century was swift
and devastating. In 1347 the bubonic plague rapidly trav-
elled westward across India and southwest Russian. The
Christian defenders may have won the day in saving Pales-
tine from the invading Ottoman Turks, but in traveling

home a majority of them died at sea. Those who managed to reach Italy started an epidemic that spread like wildfire throughout the rest of Europe. In Marseilles, France, almost 80 percent of the entire population was dead within months.

Sometime in the year 1722, a quartet of scoundrels plundered clothing, jewels, money, and other valuables from the homes and bodies of the wealthy dead. It is not known how they came up with the idea of soaking peeled and macerated garlic cloves in old wine, but that is precisely what they did. After an unspecified period of time, this aged garlic preparation was strained into stone jugs and utilized by these bandits wherever they went. They would liberally apply the stuff to their necks, faces, hands, and arms, as well as gargle and swallow sufficient quantities of it. Then they would venture out and brazenly rob the dead.

In time, their luck ran out and they were caught. But instead of being put to death, they were closely questioned by the magistrates as to how they had managed to survive while all around them were dying.

After being promised clemency from their terrible crimes, they shared the secret antidote with everyone in the courtroom. As a result, the remaining citizens of Marseilles were able to resist the plague, which soon passed from the region for good.

GERARD'S CURE FOR WORMS

The last herbal we will consider was written by John Gerard and first published in 1597. Appropriately entitled *The Herbal or General History of Plants*, it was mostly copied by Gerard from Dr. Priest's translation of an ancient herbal by Dodoens. After Priest died, Gerard plagiarized much of

this work without giving due credit to either the good doctor or the original author, so many of the remedies mentioned in Gerard's book come to us from antiquity.

Gerard, or rather Dodoens, believed that garlic was very
good for expelling intestinal parasites. If the garlic was too
overpowering, it could "be boyled in water untill such time
as it hath lost his sharpenesse" and then be more easily
tolerated in the system. "It killeth worms in the belly, and
driveth them forth," Gerard wrote.

But in order for it to be agreeable to adults and children
alike, it needed to be "boyled in milke," after which it could
then be used "with good successe against the wormes."

For getting rid of ringworm, he advised mixing a little
crushed garlic "with tempered honey, and the parts
anointed therewith."

Garlic's success for the diverse and sometimes strange
uses cited in this chapter depended on its many marvelous
constituents. By understanding something about them we
are better able to appreciate how this foul herb works in
such fabulous ways.

CHAPTER FOUR

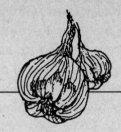

What Makes Garlic Work?

SULPHUR, AN ELEMENT WE NEED MORE OF

WITHIN the last couple of decades, several trace elements have come to the forefront in the popular and scientific literature because of what they can do to inhibit the development of cancer. These nutrients have been widely trumpeted, especially in consumer health magazines. By now, most health-conscious people recognize that selenium, germanium, and zinc can help them lower the risks of contracting cancer.

But a careful study of over 417 articles published in dozens of health magazines since 1971 failed to show even a single article devoted to the benefits of sulphur. Only in the medical and scientific journals, with their more limited circulations geared more towards academic audiences, could I find a reference to sulphur.

A couple of years ago I spoke at the Cancer Control Society convention in Los Angeles on "Sulphur Foods in the Prevention and Treatment of Cancer." I had the biggest audience of all the speakers, simply because so many people wanted to know more about this least understood and little known member of the mineral kingdom. I was barraged with questions from consumers and media people alike.

"Why don't we ever hear more about this mineral in the fight against cancer, if it's so important?" I was asked by a journalist from the *Los Angeles Times*. "What will it take to put sulphur on the health food store shelves with the other anti-cancer nutrients you just mentioned?" someone else inquired.

"They're already there in various food forms," I rejoined. "Look for your sulphur needs in blackstrap molasses (one tablespoon daily) or black mission figs (about six a day), provided you don't have blood sugar problems. Also you may find additional sulphur in dried apricots and aged garlic extract from Japan. The aging process increases sulphur content.

"And don't forget members of the Brassica family," I continued. "The work of Lee Wattenberg at the University of Minnesota School of Medicine and others elsewhere, has amply demonstrated that cabbage, kale, kohlrabi, Brussels sprouts, mustard greens, watercress, leeks, onions, radish, cauliflower, and horseradish contain different sulphur compounds which actually thwart the development of chemically-inducted tumors within the stomach and colon. In other words, those foods that have a distinct smell when they're cooked (such as cabbage), or make your eyes water when cut (such as onions), or grab your taste buds by their roots with an unmistakable pungency (like horseradish), have an abundance of sulphur."

Sulphur is an element that we just can't be without if we hope to stay free from cancer and enjoy better health!

WHAT THE SULPHUR IN GARLIC CAN DO

One expert on the chemistry of garlic, whom I met at the First World Congress on the Health Significance of Garlic and Garlic Constituents, held in Washington, D.C., in August of 1990, is Dr. Eric Block of the State University of New York at Albany. He spoke to a crowded room on "The Organic Chemistry of Garlic Sulphur Compounds." He said that "garlic unleashes at least 100 sulphur-containing compounds," all of which are linked to its wonderful medicinal uses.

"If you leave them undisturbed," he told some of us later on, "then the [garlic] bulb has very limited medicinally active compounds. But cutting it triggers the formation of a cascade of compounds that are quite reactive and that participate in a complex sequence of chemical reactions. Ultimately, an amazing collection of chemical compounds is produced."

In a more detailed article in the March 1985 issue of *Scientific American* (252:114) entitled "The Chemistry of Garlic and Onions," Dr. Block noted that many of these sulphur compounds had accomplished remarkable feats. For example, the French bacteriologist Louis Pasteur first reported in 1858 that garlic killed harmful bacteria, and in the 1950s the great humanitarian Dr. Albert Schweitzer made use of garlic's sulphur compounds for treating amoebic dysentery in many of his African patients.

Block noted that in both of the World Wars fought in this century, garlic was routinely used by military physicians as an effective antiseptic agent in the prevention of gangrene in combat wounds when penicillin was not available.

Moreover, laboratory investigations in the past few decades have proven that garlic juice diluted to a very small fraction of its strength (1:125,000) inhibits the growth of staph, strep, dysentery, and typhoid bacteria. Additionally, the same juice exhibits a broad spectrum of activity against harmful fungi and innumerable strains of yeast, including the nasty *Candida albicans,* which is responsible for thrush and vaginitis.

In some provinces of France, Dr. Block observed, race and work horses suffering from blood clots are routinely fed both garlic and onions in their grain feed. As a result, such clots dissolve within a matter of days, eliminating the apparent danger to these valuable animals.

Furthermore, in 1979 medical researchers at the B. J. College of the University of Poona in India published the results of an intensive study of three separate populations that consumed differing amounts of garlic and onions. Those being tested were members of the strictly vegetarian Jain community. Some ate lots of garlic and onions (50 grams of garlic and 600 grams of onions weekly), some ate both occasionally (usually under 10 grams of garlic and 200 grams of onions weekly), while others abstained from them altogether. Those never consuming garlic or onions had the shortest blood-coagulation time. In that group, moreover, the blood-plasma level of the blood clot forming protein fibrinogen proved to be the highest of all three groups evaluated.

I am reminded of an incident that occurred some years ago when I was in my early teens. There lived at that time in Provo, Utah, a family by the name of Young, whom we visited on a regular basis. The old grandpa, an ornery coot named Spencer Young (who was related to Brigham Young, the great Mormon colonizer) was always troubled with plugged sinuses. In order to effectively open them, he was in the habit of inhaling the sulphur fumes from a small sliver of peeled, sliced garlic, which seemed to give him considerable relief.

One time while I was visiting the family, he seemed in a highly agitated state for no apparent reason. After I made a timid inquiry into his sudden change of mood, he snapped back at this then 13-year-old lad with characteristic bluntness: "I've got this blankety-blank piece of garlic stuck up in the top of my nostril, and the blankety-blank thing just won't come out!"

He demanded that I help him in trying to extricate it from his nose. First, we tried pouring a little water up his nostril with the aid of a small funnel, but without much success. Next, he bent his head over into his lap and told me to pound on his back in the hopes it might fall out. When this didn't work, I meekly suggested tapping the back of his head with the palm of my hand, which he reluctantly assented to, but immediately screamed out his displeasure in a stream of profanities after I "accidentally" delivered a well-deserved whack against his skull. In the end, he placed one end of a vacuum hose into the inflamed nostril and sucked it out that way, but not before having endured the miseries accompanying garlic's wonderful odiferous benefits!

ANTIDOTE FOR DEADLY VENOM

In the previous chapter I discussed garlic's use for different types of bites in the Egyptian *Book of Bites* and the ancient herbal authored by Dioscorides. The work of Wattenberg and others has helped us understand at least a part of the mechanism behind this cure. The sulphur in garlic, onion, leek, and other vegetables bonds or links up with individual molecules of poison and renders them inert before they pass through the liver. A similar process is at work when sulphur compounds come between two or more chemical food additives and prevent them from linking to form potentially cancer-causing agents within the body.

It is one thing to read about garlic being used anciently for dangerous bites and stings, and quite another to see its application up front and first-hand! In early January, 1990, I attended the third symposium of the International Association for the Study of Traditional Asian Medicine (IASTAM) in Bombay. There I gave a paper on the medical relevancy of gotu kola, a common weed widespread throughout much of Southeast Asia.

One afternoon I was invited to go with an Ayurvedic physician acquaintance of mine to a local bazaar. There I was treated to an intriguing but highly dangerous snake charming exhibition put on by a scrawny looking fellow squatting in the dirt. He played his flute and moved from side to side while a huge king cobra slowly raised itself out of a reed basket directly in front of him.

Talk about living close to the edge, I thought to myself. This is just about as close as it can get! I didn't know whether to congratulate the fellow for his indomitable courage or feel sorry for his reckless stupidity. Either way, my colleague and I and the rest of the small crowd gathered a safe distance away were in for one incredible show!

About ten minutes into this "walk on the wild side," the snake charmer made too sudden a move and was instantly punished for it by a darting bite to his hand from an offended "pet." It all happened so quickly that in between two consecutive blinks of the eyes, one side of my brain was still asking the other side, "Did you see that?" Without losing so much as a beat in the tempo of his swaying motions, the fellow, who by now had stopped playing his instrument, slowly raised his injured right hand to his mouth and deposited a curious-looking mixture of saliva and chewed vegetable matter onto his wound. Then he went back to his same deadly business of entertaining us for a few rupees tossed his way with an air of indifference to what had just occurred.

When this sinister act had concluded and my heartbeat was back to normal, we went over to interrogate the fellow about what he had used to treat his injured hand. Acting as my interpreter, the doctor with me made the necessary inquiry, whereupon the other fellow drew out a small, dirty object from within the folds of his soiled loin cloth and, holding it aloft, exclaimed in Hindi, "Lasan! Lasan!" Which meant "Garlic! Garlic!" He then showed us how he methodically chewed a clove before giving a performance in case the cobra didn't appreciate his music or fast moves.

I haven't yet experimented with the same on my ranch in southern Utah, where sidewinder rattlesnakes are as plentiful as seagulls at a city landfill, but now I am convinced that this remedy really works!

While attending the World Garlic Congress I had a chance encounter with an Australian chap by the name of David C. Douglas. He was there with his small crew interviewing various speakers for a television documentary entitled "The Gift of The Gods: The Vital History and Multiple Uses of Garlic." I told him about my encounter with the Indian snake charmer. Mr. Douglas was fascinated, called his crew together, and shot a segment of me retelling the experience in the spacious lobby of the historic Willard Hotel, located next door to the White House.

The documentary was later shown on Australian television and was seen on the BBC (British Broadcasting Corporation) television network as well. Lady Edith Grayson of Suffolk County, England, wrote me a gracious letter in some of the most beautiful penmanship I've ever seen. She had watched my brief interview in the documentary and had tried the remedy herself.

Details of her experience were somewhat sketchy, but this is the story she told. She had been outside doing some weeding in her back estate garden when a snake of some unknown species and considered to be fairly poisonous bit her on the finger. She remembered what I had said about the snake charmer and went into her kitchen, peeled a clove of garlic and began hurriedly to chew it. She applied this mixture to her wound, gently rubbing it into the two puncture marks left by the snake's fangs. She then lay down for awhile and claimed this made her feel much better. According to her, she suffered no ill effects after this.

Now I've employed crushed garlic cloves and water in treating things such as red ant bites and wasp strings with good success. I even had a case once where I administered warm garlic and onion tea to a teenager who was suffering from the effects of a hornet sting by hyperventilating and profusely sweating. Within 30 minutes her breathing, pulse rate, and perspiration returned to normal.

If the Indian snake charmer is correct, it may be that the sulphur compounds in garlic are just as effective in neutralizing deadly snake venom as they are for insect and chemical toxins.

NUTRITIONAL GOODNESS IN A SINGLE CLOVE

Another speaker at the World Garlic Conference was Dr. Yoichi Itakura of the Wakunaga Pharmaceutical Co. in Hiroshima, Japan. Dr. Itakura showed his audience a series of slides, one of which listed the following general ingredients for 100 grams (edible portions) of garlic:

Water	61.3%
Carbohydrate	30.8g
Protein	6.2g
Fiber	1.5g
Fat	0.2g
Ash	1.5g
Potassium	259.0mg
Phosphorus	202.0mg
Calcium	29.0mg
Sodium	19.0mg
Iron	1.5mg
Ascorbic acid	15.0mg
Niacin	0.5mg
Thiamine	0.25mg
Riboflavin	0.08mg
Vitamin A	trace

According to Dr. Itakura, the nutrients in aged garlic provided energy and stamina to a number of volunteers on whom it was tested. To briefly summarize his scientific paper, he observed that in clinical studies with 1,000 patients, aged garlic extract demonstrated remarkable anti-fatigue activity, which he attributed to its sulphur components.

Other scientists have discovered additional trace elements as well. The proven anticancer nutrient germanium, mentioned earlier, is one of them. According to *Chemical & Pharmaceutical Bulletin* (28:2691, 1980), the following herbs contain these amounts of germanium (in parts per billion or ppb):

GERMANIUM

Garlic bulb	1 ppb
Ginseng root (3 g)	5 ppb
Comfrey leaf	1 ppb
Comfrey root	2 ppb

The April 1989 edition of *Deutsche Zeitschrift für Onkologie* (German *Journal of Oncology*) mentioned other specific nutrients in garlic in an excellent article titled, "Enhancement of Natural Killer Cell Activity in AIDS with Garlic." According to the article, "Therapeutic factors in garlic include ... magnesium, selenium, [and] 17 amino acids. ... Garlic is one of the richest sources of organic selenium and germanium." Together, garlic's disclosed and yet undiscovered nutrients combine to make it one of the best nutritional food spices in the world.

WHAT'S CURRENT AND PASSÉ IN GARLIC CHEMISTRY

Because garlic has so many different compounds, it would be impossible within a work this size to do them all justice. As Dr. Block correctly stated, "The deeper you look into garlic's wonderful chemistry, the more you tend to discover what you didn't know before." As those of us who went to Japan in 1990 quickly learned, this strange and intriguing chemistry can take even more fascinating twists and turns when garlic undergoes a cold aging process.

Following are some of garlic's less known but equally medically relevant compounds. Clearly, there is a lot more to garlic than what may meet the eye or greet the nose and palate.

ADENOSINE 'THINS' THE BLOOD

Two researchers at the George Washington School of Medicine in the District of Columbia have identified a common chemical substance shared by garlic and onion which is the primary blocker of blood platelet clumping in allium vegetables. It is called adenosine and is not destroyed by cooking. Drs. Amar Makheja and John M. Bailey claim that raw and cooked garlic and onions can help "thin" the blood in much the same way that ginger root does, thereby warding off potentially dangerous clots.

Adenosine also occurs in scallions (green bunching onions) and shallots (garlic-shaped bulbs with tissue-wrapped cloves that taste more like onion than garlic and are often used in French cooking).

ALLICIN WONDERLAND

When I think of all the marketing hype some garlic companies have given this ephemeral sulphur compound, I'm reminded of Alice in Wonderland, a world in which "nothing is as it seems and yet everything is as it seems."

This sums up the arguments put forth about allicin. Some manufacturers contend that allicin is an effective antibiotic substance, which makes their particular brands superior. But in the highly competitive health food industry, where fact and fiction often get mixed together, consumers need to heed the Latin maxim *Caveat emptor* ("Let the buyer beware").

Here is the low-down on allicin, plain and simple. When garlic is crushed or sliced, an odorless and flavorless compound known as alliin makes contact with an enzyme called allinase, and together they create allicin, a compound first isolated in garlic in 1944. But, as Drs. Eric Block and Yoichi Itakura reiterated at the First World Congress on Garlic, "allicin is *very, very* unstable," to say the least. Studies show that, in pure form, its half-life is less than three hours. Dr. Itakura observed that "in organic solvents, allicin disappears in a day at room temperature." Dr. Block informed me in private conversation that "allicin may last for a couple of days if you refrigerate it at a sufficiently cold temperature," but after that it's history, chemically speaking.

Even when vegetable or citrus oils are added as stabilizers to garlic products that brag about their purported allicin contents, the effect only lasts a week or so, noted Dr. Willis R. Brewer, a pharmacognosist and Dean and Professor Emeritus in the College of Pharmacy at the University of Arizona. "Many of the claims based on allicin are out of date, misleading, and in some cases untrue," he wrote. "Allicin is a mispromoted substance. Allicin," he concluded, "is not a suitable substance for the standardization of garlic products."

His and Drs. Block's and Itakura's conclusions about the near worthlessness of allicin is supported by many other scientists. For instance, Drs. Neil Caporaso, Sharon M. Smith, and Robert H. K. Eng, writing in the May 1983 issue of *Antimicrobial Agents and Chemotherapy*, concluded that "allicin has *limited* potential as an oral therapy ..." Furthermore, even *if* adequate allicin were able to get into the body, it would still be "weakened through reduction and in the presence of blood," wrote Dr. Bep Oliver-Bever in *Medicinal Plants in Tropical West Africa* (London: Cambridge University Press, 1986; p. 135).

Unless you're into health food fairy tales, don't be persuaded that just because a particular garlic product *claims* it contains significant amounts of allicin, this makes it superior to others without it. To paraphrase Lewis Carroll, "allicin is there, but then and again, it isn't."

Allixin, A Wonderful Anti-Stress Compound

When Earl Mindell, Morton Walker and I joined some of our European colleagues in Hiroshima, Japan, in 1991, we were the first to be introduced to an exciting new sulphur compound which had just then been isolated from aged garlic by Dr. Y. Kodera and his team at the Wakunaga Pharmaceutical Co. They named it *allixin.*

Some plants are known to produce stress compounds. When a normal living plant tissue is injured by the attack of chemical or physical stress, important data is rapidly transmitted from the injured tissue through a plant's neural network to another normal tissue. Then the informed normal tissue begins production of abnormal substances called "stress compounds." Some of these stress compounds have anti-microbial properties and are called *phytoalexins* (phyto = plant, alexin = to ward off).

There are major weapons for plant defense. Well known examples include rishitin (produced by members of the nightshade family such as tomatoes, potatoes, and tobacco), glyceollin (produced by soybeans) and pisatin (produced by garden peas). Since many of these phytoalexins are induced by exposure of a plant to bacteria, viruses, fungi, ultraviolet rays, or heavy metal salts, they can serve as powerful disinfectants against disease processes in the human body.

This is also the case with allixin. According to a report in *Cancer Letters* (59:89–90, 1991), this newly discovered garlic compound "significantly reduces" the promoting of a particular chemical carcinogen on tumor development in general. Therefore, when we speak of allixin as being an anti-stress compound, we don't mean it in the same way that herbal sedatives like valerian, hops, or catnip are understood. Allixin reduces the infection stresses imposed upon the body by disease itself.

It would probably be more correct to say that allixin is an *anti-disease* rather than an anti-stress compound. When you include garlic in your diet more frequently, you are actually *preventing* any number of disease processes, and the evidence seems to suggest that the more the garlic is stressed (chopped, minced, pressed), the more allixin there is to be found in it.

PREVENTING BLOOD CLOTS WITH AJOENE

Dr. Eric Block has been one of the principal researchers involved in the discovery and isolation of a medically important sulphur compound called ajoene (pronounced ay-HO-een). His work in the early 1970s was expanded upon by scientists from the University of Delaware and the Venezuelan Institute of Scientific Investigations in Caracas. They were able to produce several garlic extracts that were especially aggressive in preventing the clumping of blood platelets. In close collaboration with their other colleagues, Dr. Block and Saleem Ahmad established the chemical structure of this new compound. "We named the compound ajoene, after *ajo* (pronounced aho), Spanish for garlic," he wrote in the March 1985 issue of *Scientific American*.

Ajoene, they found, is formed by self-condensation from allicin. Clinical experiments have shown that as a potential antithrombotic agent, it is just as effective as plain aspirin. Studies by the Delaware and Venezuela groups, in collaboration with James Catalfamo of the New York State Department of Health in Albany, suggest that ajoene acts by inhibiting fibrinogen receptors on platelets. Further work is currently underway to see how useful ajoene may be as an anticoagulant drug.

AJOENE WORKS AGAINST FUNGI AND CANCER

A group of Japanese scientists from the Central Research Laboratories of Wakunaga Pharmaceutical in Hiroshima, tested six different sulphur fractions derived from garlic in an in vitro (cultured media) system. Only ajoene showed the strongest activity against two types of fungi, *Aspergillus niger* (often present in the outer ear canal) and *Candida albicans* (responsible for oral thrush and vaginitis). This report appeared in the March 1987 issue of *Applied and Environmental Microbiology*.

The August 1991 *Harvard Health Letter* noted that ajoene "is toxic to Burkitt's lymphoma cells when they are grown in tissue culture." Other sulphur compounds within garlic "will block the development of colon, esophageal, and skin cancers in rodents exposed to specific chemical carcinogens that produce these malignancies," the report continued. And lab rodents, into which fresh bladder tumors were directly transplanted, experienced no further growth of them when fed aged garlic extract.

Epidemiological studies conducted in the Shandong province of China, where stomach cancer is quite prevalent, and in Italy, have shown that garlic consumers rate 60 percent lower in this type of malignancy than those who don't eat garlic or other allium vegetables like onions, chives, and scallions. (*Diet, Life-style and Mortality in China: A Study of the*

Characteristics of 65 Chinese Counties by C. Junshi, T. Colin
Campbell, L. Junyao, and R. Peto, was published in 1990 by
Cornell University Press, Ithaca, New York.)

This leads one to ask, "Can garlic-gorging effectively
treat cancer in humans?" The jury is still out, but of one
thing we can be certain: regular garlic consumption does
prevent the formation of cancer in a number of cases.

PECTINS ARE GOOD FOR CHOLESTEROL REDUCTION

The outer skins of garlic and onion contain a great
deal of pectin. This is a gelatinous fiber found in all fruits
and most vegetables. Therapeutically, pectin has been used
to control diarrhea (often in conjunction with other agents),
as a blood plasma expander, and, more recently, as an agent
to lower serum cholesterol and triglycerides in the blood
and liver. Further information on the role of pectin in garlic
appears in the scientific literature.

S-ALLYL-CYSTEINE REDUCES "BAD" CHOLESTEROL

Studies carried out on cholesterol-sensitive hens at
the University of Wisconsin in Madison several years ago
showed that another sulphur compound in garlic can reduce
"bad" cholesterol (low-density lipoproteins or LDL). In
chickens given either aged garlic extract or S-allyl-cysteine,
LDL-cholesterol was reduced by as much as 50 percent.
Plasma triglycerides, now implicated more in ateriosclerosis
than LDL used to be, were also substantially lowered.

DIALLYL TRISULFIDE (DAST) IS LIVER FRIENDLY AND ANTIVIRAL

During the processing and aging of garlic, several other unique compounds are formed. They are the diallyl sulfide group, consisting of diallyl sulfide, diallyl disulfide and diallyl trisulfide, the last two having two and three sulphur molecules, respectively. Our focus here is with the last of these, diallyl trisulfide. It is very friendly to the liver and helps this organ perform its many functions better.

Meningitis is an infection of the three membranes, called the meninges, that lie between the brain and the skull. It can be contagious and is induced by poor nutrition and any number of viruses (such as poliomyelitis and measles), fungi (such as yeast), or bacteria (including pneumoccus and tuberculosis).

A report from the Hunan Medical College in mainland China in 1980 told of 11 cases of human cryptococcal meningitis being successfully treated with garlic extract. The garlic extract was given orally plus either intramuscularly or intravenously over a period of nearly a month. Side effects were minimal, including transient chills, low-grade fever, headache, nausea, vomiting, and pain at the injection sites.

Some years later, as more became known about diallyl trisulfide, I remembered this incident and mentioned it to one of the scientists I met during a trip to Japan. While his name has slipped my mind, what he said has not. I asked him if diallyl trisulfide might have been a key factor in killing the particular yeast-like fungi that had infected the nervous systems and brains of these eleven patients. He pointed out that garlic has many different sulphur compounds capable of antibiotic action but agreed that diallyl trisulfide could have done more than most of the others due to its remarkable antifungal and antibacterial strength.

TEAMWORK AMONG THE SULPHUR COMPOUNDS

This chapter was never intended to be a comprehensive text on the fascinating chemistry of garlic—that would take an entire book all by itself. But this brief overview of some of the more important constituents gives readers a fair idea of what is involved when the amazing chemical powers of garlic are finally unleashed.

Earlier, it was mentioned that garlic has over 100 known sulphur compounds. To some scientists' way of thinking, that's just the tip of the iceberg. They believe there could be well over 500 different compounds waiting to be discovered in the next 50 years or so.

So far we know that many of these individual sulphur compounds help to reduce blood pressure and blood sugar, relieve asthma and bronchitis, improve circulation and heart function, prevent cancer and many other diseases, and assist the body in getting rid of dangerous toxins. Compounds that haven't even been mentioned here, such as scordinin or steroidal glycosides, or barely treated in passing, like selenium, are responsible for some of these actions.

I am reminded of something a friend once told me, that puts everything relating to garlic's magnificent chemistry into proper perspective. Mas Ohkubo said; "What makes garlic so effective is not alliin, not allicin, not ajoene, but a *combined* effect of over 100 different compounds."

The many different chemical components in garlic are like a lavish buffet. No individual item constitutes the entire spread, but taken together, all the entrees provide balanced nourishment and remedial assistance to hungry bodies in need of rejuvenation. That's the way garlic works to improve your health!

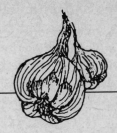

CHAPTER FIVE

Garlic Therapy in Disease Management

DOCUMENTING THE EVIDENCE

BEFORE going on to Chapter Six which is devoted to the wide variety of garlic preparations and how each may be effectively used, what follows here is pertinent information for a whole range of health problems, including which form of garlic therapy might be the most appropriate.

What about the effectiveness of the different forms of garlic on the market? As Dr. Subhuti Dharmananda, Director of the Institute for Traditional Medicine and Preventive Health Care in Portland, Oregon, observed in his article on commercial garlic supplements in the September/October 1991 issue of *Body, Mind and Spirit* magazine: "There has been much more clinical research and medical experience with the Japanese and European brands (Kyolic, Katsu, and Kwai) than with the American brands . . ." In fact, anybody caring to survey the published research on garlic between 1982 and 1992 in the MEDLARS or MEDLINE computer systems established by the National Library of Medicine in Bethesda, Maryland, will quickly discover that a *full 65 percent* or better was done using Japanese aged garlic extract (JAGE). Another 15 percent of the research used European manufactured garlic (EMG), while the remaining 20 percent utilized only raw garlic (RG).

Therefore, whenever a piece of research is briefly presented, instead of mentioning the particular brand which was used, I will refer to one of these three generic categories instead, either by the full name or its respective abbreviation: Japanese aged garlic extract (JAGE), European manufactured garlic (EMG), or raw garlic (RG). This way the reader will know which form of garlic scientists used in their clinical tests and laboratory experiments. This does not mean that American manufactured garlic isn't of some use; it just means that those in the scientific world have shown a decided preference for JAGE, EMG or RG in their research.

ACNE

Dr. Harold Simons, formerly of Duluth, Minnesota, told me at a major health convention in Chicago that he has always prescribed garlic for his young adult patients suffering from acne. While the ideal would be to include four cloves of garlic every day in the diet, this isn't always practical, especially with young people, who might shun garlic because of its odor. Therefore, he has recommended eight (EMG) tablets or four capsules daily, as well as bathing existing eruptions in a garlic infusion or liniment. A handy lotion that he recommends calls for eight fluid ounces of rubbing alcohol mixed with one and a half ounces of freshly made garlic paste (see Chapter Six under "Packing"). Stir the mixture well and keep it refrigerated. This can be dabbed on at regular intervals with a pair of cotton Q-tips held together. The liquid dries out the skin and helps to unclog blocked pores preventing them from becoming infected.

AIDS

In 1986 two microbiologists from Loma Linda University School of Medicine in Loma Linda, California, published a paper showing that dehydrated garlic powder made from fresh garlic bulbs inhibited the growth and evolution of the medically important dimorphic fungus, *Coccidioides immitis*, which usually infects patients suffering from AIDS (*Current Microbiology* 13:73–76, 1986).

Two other reports of great significance show how valuable garlic can be in treating this ever expanding worldwide epidemic. Laurence Badgley, M.D., of Foster City, California, has treated hundreds of AIDS and ARC (AIDS-related cases) patients in the last decade. In his book *Healing AIDS Naturally* (San Bruno, CA: Human Energy Press, 1987), he referred to one patient who suffered from Kaposi sarcoma (common to full-blown AIDS cases) plus numerous other symptoms. Part of the program he was placed on included "approximately eight to nine cloves of raw garlic ... each day" and "increasing his vitamin C to 60–80 grams per day, taken with lemon and honey in a drink, all with a good effect," Badgley wrote.

In 1988 doctors at the Akbar Clinic and Research Foundation in Panama City, Florida, undertook a pilot study treating ten AIDS patients with Japanese aged garlic extract (JAGE) for a period of three months. Five grams of JAGE were taken daily during the first six weeks and ten grams were taken daily for the second six weeks. Three patients died within the experimental period, leaving seven to complete the regimen. As reported in the German medical journal *Deutsche Zeitschrift für Onkologie* (2:52–53, April 1989), they experienced enhancement of natural killer cell activity and improvement of some of their other AIDS symptoms, such as diarrhea, genital herpes, candidiasis, and pansinusitis.

ARTERIOSCLEROSIS AND ATHEROSCLEROSIS

The difference between these two illnesses has always been confusing. The first, arteriosclerosis, concerns the buildup of calcium deposits on the inside of artery walls, which causes thickening and hardening of the arteries. The second, atherosclerosis, exists when these deposits are fatty substances instead. Both conditions have the same effect on circulation in that they can cause strokes, angina, and hypertension.

R. C. Jain, M.D., with the Department of Pathology at the University of Benghazi in Libya, reported on the "significant" effects that garlic, but not onion, had in reducing cholesterol levels and atherosclerosis in cholesterol-fed rabbits in the British Medical journal *The Lancet* (May 31, 1975, p. 1240). The same study in greater detail appeared in *Artery* (1:115–125, 1975). Raw garlic in distilled water was used.

David Kritchevsky of the Wistar Institute of Anatomy and Biology in Philadelphia reported in *Artery* (1:319–23, 1975) that garlic oil achieved the same results with cholesterol-fed rabbits. Dr. Jain and his colleague, D. B. Konar, duplicated Kritchevsky's work with similar results (*The Lancet*, April 24, 1976, p. 918).

G. Sainani, D. B. Desai, and K. N. More studied three groups of healthy people from the Jain community in India. The first group made liberal use of garlic and onion in their diets; the second group never used these herbs at all; and the third group, who were blood relatives of the second group, used small amounts of garlic and onion occasionally. The first and last groups registered very little or no atherosclerosis, while the middle group, who used no raw garlic or onion, registered enormously higher serum triglycerides, beta-lipoprotein, phospholipids, plasma fibrinogen values, and serum cholesterol—all important markers of atherosclerosis (*The Lancet*, 1976, no. 7985, pp. 575–76).

Reuters news agency in London reported on June 6, 1978, that West German scientists in Cologne had been able to reduce atherosclerosis in volunteers fed butter with garlic oil capsules (EMG) and raw garlic. Other volunteers, who consumed butter without the benefit of either form of garlic, registered much higher serum cholesterol levels and more of the atherosclerotic process.

The team of Jain and Konar conducted still another experiment with cholesterol-fed male albino rabbits, which was reported in *Atherosclerosis* (29:125–29, 1978). This time they administered garlic juice, which greatly inhibited atherogenesis in the rabbit aortas.

Benjamin Lau, M.D., and two others from Loma Linda University Schools of Medicine and Health did a review of the published research on garlic and atherosclerosis up to 1982 (*Nutrition Research* 3:119–28, 1983). The majority of reports were very favorable in supporting garlic therapy for the prevention and treatment of atherosclerosis. "The majority of the published data," they observed, "suggest a dose-related effect of garlic." JAGE and RG were used in the studies they surveyed.

In *Agricultural and Biological Chemistry* (49:1187–88, 1985) the presence of certain polyunsaturated fatty acids normally found in fish were discovered in garlic as well. Two of them in particular, arachidonic and eicosapentaenoic acids, were believed to explain garlic's role in controlling atherosclerosis. Raw garlic was used.

The New York Times (Tuesday, September 4, 1990) reported on the results of an interesting three-year study conducted in Udaipur, India, by cardiologist Arun Bordia, M.D., of the Tagore Medical College. He randomly divided 432 coronary patients who had already suffered one heart attack into two groups, one of which received daily supplements of garlic juice in milk. Those who took the garlic suffered fewer additional heart attacks, had lower blood pressure and serum cholesterol levels, and were less likely to die during the study. After three years, nearly twice as many patients had died in the group not taking garlic. Dr. Bordia explained that the benefits of garlic became increasingly apparent with time, suggesting that the herb worked by dissolving the atherosclerotic blockages in coronary arteries. Raw garlic was used.

This study, as well as several others, demonstrates that garlic can not only prevent but even *reverse* the early stages of atherosclerosis. The best forms of garlic therapy for this would be anything that is liquid: garlic essence (one tablespoon daily); encapsulated oil (four daily); fluid extract (one teaspoon daily); raw juice (one quarter teaspoon in one half cup goat's milk); tea (one half cup twice daily); tincture (30 drops daily); or wine (two tablespoons daily). See Chapter Six for directions for preparing these garlic products.

ARTHRITIS

The *Yomiuri Shimbun*, one of Tokyo's largest newspapers, carried a story in April of 1980 describing research that tested Japanese aged garlic extract on patients suffering from arthritis and lumbago. The treatment showed an 86 percent improvement with no adverse side effects. An American physician, William H. Khoe, M.D., reported in his *Khoe Newsletter* that he recommended JAGE (up to 10 capsules daily) to all of his arthritis patients for relief of their pain and reduction of their joint swellings with good results. Garlic does this by curbing the activity of free radicals, which cause considerable tissue damage. (See page 96-98 for more data.)

BITES

See pages 37-38, 45, 54-56 and 114 for information on garlic treatment for bites.

BLOOD CLOTS

Dr. Bordia's previously cited work with the Jain community in India demonstrated that garlic dramatically increased the fibrinolytic activity of the blood. That's a fancy way of saying garlic splits up or dissolves a protein (called fibrin) that is essential to blood clot formation. Those who have heart disease or varicose veins may be at risk for getting blood clots. Because a diseased heart pumps blood less vigorously, blood flow may be slowed. This increases the chance of a clot forming in the heart. Varicose veins also tend to slow blood flow, leading to formation of a clot in a leg vein. This is why natural blood thinners such as garlic, ginger root, or cayenne pepper are important to take on a regular basis.

Those most at risk from blood clots are usually the middle-aged and elderly, those who are somewhat obese and physically inactive, and those who have irregular heart rate (atrial fibrillation), an artificial heart valve, heart valve disease, atherosclerosis, or thrombophlebitis in the legs. They need the benefits of garlic the most to prevent blood clots from occurring.

The garlic compound ajoene is as potent as aspirin in preventing sticky red blood platelets from clumping together. Several papers on ajoene were given at the 1990 World Garlic Congress in Washington, D.C., by scientists from the University of Caracas in Venezuela and the University of Delaware.

Still another aspirin-like component in garlic that helps to "thin" the blood is allicin—one of the odiferous but highly unstable compounds. Dr. Krishna Agrawal, professor of pharmacology at Tulane University, has found that it, too, stops platelets from clumping.

The Orlando Sentinel (Thursday, August 2, 1990, p. H-6) reported that Dr. John Martyn Bailey of George Washington University School of Medicine identified another component of garlic and onion, adenosine, as being a "blood-thinning" agent. Chinese black mushrooms called "three ears" are rich in adenosine and are anticoagulants. In the studies previously mentioned, an alcohol extract of raw garlic and raw garlic itself were used.

Dr. David J. Bouillin's report in *The Lancet* (1:776–77, 1981) showed that garlic was an effective platelet inhibitor. Working at the Clinical Pharmacology Research Unit in Oxford, England, he gave volunteers four raw cloves each and found that, an hour later, their blood had totally lost its ability to stick together; this ability gradually returned over two and a half hours as the garlic substances were lost or excreted. Concerned that his original dose didn't realistically reflect people's eating habits, he repeated the experiments using normal English dietary amounts, no more than a third of a clove over two daily meals. He looked for volunteers who had never consumed garlic, but so set were people's tastes that nobody would take him up on his daring offer. So he put together a group of garlic eaters, took them off their favorite spice for 30 days, and then gave them the smaller doses. He found that their blood was significantly less sticky for the same length of time and concluded that daily use of garlic will alter the blood's long-term tendency to clot.

More recently, a new synthetic garlic molecule, which retains the herb's anti-clotting ability, has been patented by Dr. Robert Hermes, a polymer scientist at the Los Alamos National Laboratory in New Mexico. He managed to unite the various sulphide compounds in garlic that prevent clotting with a plastic molecule, which he hopes can be eventually used to coat the lining of artificial hearts and arteries to prevent bacteria from growing where low blood flow is apt to cause clots to form.

All of the liquid garlic preparations mentioned at the end of ARTERIOSCLEROSIS (page 72) in the amounts given would be helpful for preventing blood clots, as would the use of garlic tablets (five daily) and the frequent use of raw garlic in meal preparations.

BOILS & CYSTS

A registered nurse who attended one of my health lectures in Chicago in 1992 told me what she did to get rid of boils and cysts in some of her patients. She cut a piece of an old, clean linen sheet into an oblong measuring about one by two inches. She soaked this with olive oil and wrung out the excess, then crushed one peeled garlic clove very fine and spread it over half of the cloth to make a crude paste. She then folded over the other half of the linen to make the crushed clove into an inch square sandwich. She taped this directly over the boil or cyst and changed the dressing every day. She said that this not only helped to relieve the pain and inflammation, it also broke down the plug blocking the sebaceous duct very quickly. Sometimes she would apply some medicated petroleum jelly around the swelling to insure that the pad only came in contact with the erupting head of the infected area.

BREAST-FEEDING PROBLEMS

Science News (140:230, Oct. 12, 1991) reported that breast-fed babies drink more vigorously and consume more milk after their mothers consumed garlic, as compared to babies of non-garlic eating moms. Also, the October 1991 issue of the journal *Pediatrics* reported that "during feed periods when the milk smelled most strongly of garlic, the infants were attached to the breast longer and drank more milk." Nursing mothers are, therefore, encouraged to eat more raw garlic. Odorless supplements won't work in this case.

BURNS

See pages 38-42.

CANCER

Much information has been derived from a variety of biochemical, biological, clinical, environmental, epidemiological, or nutritional studies to show that garlic can prevent cancer. A condensed survey of some of this literature follows.

Japanese scientists at Tokushima University made an analysis of garlic bulb, ginseng root, comfrey root and leaf, and green tea leaves, among other plants, and discovered minute traces of the anticancer nutrient germanium, which they measured in ppb (parts per billion) units (*Chemical and Pharmaceutical Bulletin* 28:2687–91, 1980). The table below gives the values of germanium content for each herb:

GERMANIUM

Garlic bulb	1 ppb
Ginseng root	5–6 ppb
Comfrey root	1 ppb
Comfrey leaf	2 ppb
Green tea leaf	9 ppb

One Japanese medical doctor, who practices traditional kanpo (or kampo) medicine in addition to allopathic medicine in a cosmopolitan hospital in Tokyo, routinely prescribes for his cancer patients Japanese aged garlic extract in liquid form (four tablespoons daily) and five to six cups of warm green tea with meals. He also has them drink a ginseng root tonic made in Korea. He believes that from these three herbs they are getting the maximum amount of germanium needed to cause regression of their tumors. For further information on kanpo medicine, see Margaret M. Lock's *East Asian Medicine in Urban Japan*, Part 3 (Berkeley: University of California Press, 1980).

Dr. Mei Xing of the Shandong Province Medical College was puzzled as to why residents from Gangshan County had one of the lowest stomach cancer rates (3.4/100,000), while those in neighboring Quixia County had one of the highest (40/100,000). So he and his medical staff evaluated the dietary histories of 564 patients with the disease and compared them with those of 1,131 controls who were free of it.

He discovered, much to his amazement, that folks in Gangshan County consumed an average of 20 grams (about

¾ oz.) of allium vegetables every day, while residents in Quixia County ate very little if any garlic, garlic stalks, onions, Chinese chives, or scallions with their meals. When the subjects were grouped according to how much of these vegetables they consumed, those in the top quarter had a 60 percent lower risk of gastric cancer than those in the bottom quarter. A similar study undertaken in Italy at about the same time showed that there, too, people who ate the most garlic had an appreciably lower risk of stomach cancer (*Medical Tribune*, August 12, 1981, and *Harvard Health Letter*, August 1991).

A massive study entitled *Diet, Life-style and Mortality in China*, published in 1990 by Oxford and Cornell University Presses, evaluated the diets and lifestyles of 6,500 individuals belonging to 1,950 families in 65 of China's 2,000 counties. This nationwide survey spanned 1973–1984. The study showed that those who consumed the most sulphur-rich vegetables—such as Chinese and common cabbages, Chinese leek and garlic, mustard leaves, radish and radish leaf, and rape—had the lowest risks of cancer in general.

The book also reports that daily intakes of plant fiber, total vitamin A derivatives (carotenoids), and vitamin C, all known to have strong anticancer activity, were much higher in Chinese diets as compared to American diets. On the other hand, total daily fat and protein intakes were measurably lower for the Chinese than for the American diets. The accompanying table gives the values for each:

DIETARY INTAKES	CHINA	U.S.
Total dietary fiber (g/day)	33.3	11.1
Starch (g/day)	371	120
Plant protein (% of total protein)	89	30

DIETARY INTAKES	CHINA	U.S.
Fat (% of calories)	14.5	38.8
Calcium (mg/day)	544	1143
Retinol (vitamin A equiv/day)[1]	27.8	990
Total carotenoids (total vitamin A equiv/day)[2]	836	429
Vitamin C (mg/day)	140	73
PLASMA CONSTITUENTS		
Cholesterol (mg/dl)[3]	127	212
Triglycerides (md/dl)	97	120
Total protein (g/dl)[4]	4.8–6.2	6.4–8.3

[1]Beta-carotene levels higher in U.S., because of higher rice and grain consumptions in China.

[2]Several hundred carotenoids are now known to exist, of which beta-carotene (retinol) is the best known. Still, the Chinese intake is much higher for total vitamin A intake than it is for the U.S.

[3]Signifies cholesterol milligrams per blood deciliter.

[4]Signifies protein grams per blood deciliter.

What all of this suggests is that for the prevention of cancer in general, regular consumption of sulphur-rich vegetables, including garlic, is to be strongly encouraged.

The *St. Petersburg Evening Independent* (March 24, 1986) reported on separate research in New York and Texas showing that 1,200 milligrams of calcium carbonate and Japanese aged garlic extract (2 capsules) would inhibit colon cancer.

Benjamin Lau, M.D., Ph.D. of Loma Linda School of Medicine, who has become one of the leading garlic researchers in the world, told me how he first became interested in the spice. "As I was visiting a physician friend in his home, he told me that he had used garlic preparations in his practice and that his patients had enjoyed relief from a variety of complaints. In the course of our conversation, he mentioned that garlic is a potent antibiotic and inhibitor of many germs. As a professor of microbiology, I began devising in my mind a test to find out if my friend was right. At the time, my students and I were doing experiments testing the activity of several new antibiotics on bacteria and fungi. Upon returning to my laboratory, I prepared a diluted garlic extract, introduced a small quantity into several cultures and let them incubate overnight. The next day I was astounded to find that the diluted garlic extract did indeed stop the growth of those cultures—more effectively, in fact, than some of the potent antibiotics we were testing at that time."

Dr. Lau said that this discovery prompted him to do a search through the scientific literature to see if any research had ever been done on garlic and tumors. He eventually discovered such a report published in *Science* journal (126:1112–14, November 29, 1957), over 35 years ago, in which researchers at Western Reserve University had used raw garlic enzyme (alliinase) to prevent the growth of sarcoma in Swiss mice by inactivating certain chemical components of these tumor cells called sulfhydryl compounds. In time he switched from raw garlic to JAGE, believing that it was more potent and could demonstrate greater antitumor activity with considerably fewer side-effects than raw garlic has. More recently, he compared Japanese aged garlic extract with three additional garlic extracts obtained from local health food stores in the southern California area, in immune stimulation. He and his colleagues, Drs. Takeshi Yamasaki and Daila S. Gridley, noticed that JAGE significantly enhanced the fighting ability of a macrophage cell line whereas the other unidentified garlic supplements did not. Macrophages are an important part of the body's immune defenses. This research appeared in *Molecular Biotherapy* (3:103–7, June 1991).

Dr. Lau was one of only a handful of privileged scientists who were invited by the National Cancer Institute to make recommendations for fruits, vegetables, and herbs which could be studied in their new Designer Foods Research Project. Dr. Lau proposed that garlic be one of these foods, along with flaxseed, licorice root, citrus fruits, cruciferous vegetables (cabbage, broccoli, and kale), umbelliferous vegetables (celery, parsley, parsnips, and carrots), soy, and green tea. In 1992, the project's first full year of research, activities included feeding trials in animals to establish safety, and in healthy humans to determine effects of the foods on cancer-related biochemical pathways—that is, their effects on the metabolism of prostaglandins, steroids, and drugs (*Journal of the National Cancer Institute*, August 7, 1991).

Additional research by other scientists around the world has supported Lau's contention that garlic is one of the best weapons in the arsenal of natural drugs against cancer. Japanese researchers from Kyoto reported that JAGE suppressed the first stage of tumor promotion in a two-stage mouse skin cancer (*Oncology* 46:277–80, 1989). Even scientists from the National Cancer Institute and the American Cancer Society teamed up to publish a very favorable literature review of garlic's wonderful anti-cancer properties (*Preventive Medicine* 19:346–61, May 1990).

Finally, at the World Garlic Congress held in 1990 in Washington, D.C., important papers presented by American and Japanese scientists, most of whom used JAGE in their experiments showed without a doubt that garlic is effective in the prevention and treatment of cancers of the breast, stomach, colon, bladder, and skin.

From the evidence given here, it is suggested that garlic be used occasionally in raw form and frequently in capsule, tablet, fluid extract, and tincture forms to avoid as well as treat cancer.

CANDIDA

More controversy surrounds candidiasis and hypoglycemia than any other health problems I know of. On one side of the medical establishment are the firmly entrenched doctors who continue to tell patients that chronic candidiasis syndrome (a yeast infection caused by *Candida albicans*) is all in their heads. On the other side are doctors such as Tennessee allergist William G. Crook, M.D., who wrote a best-selling book entitled *The Yeast Connection* (Jackson, TN: Professional Books, 1987) which sold almost a million copies. In it he summarized his experiences with hundreds of Candida patients.

Lutretia Starr of Hayward, California related the following episode to me back in 1978: "At the beginning of July I suffered two days with a yeast infection. I took a clove of fresh garlic, put it in the blender with four ounces of water, and liquified it. I then strained the mixture through some close-woven cheese cloth. Adding enough water to make 24 ounces, I douched with eight ounces every night before bedtime, for three nights. On the fourth night I douched with a cooled tea (room temperature) made from oat straw. Little by little the terrible itching subsided. By the fourth night it was gone and by the fifth night it was completely cleared up. Isn't it wonderful to heal naturally?"

Calvin L. Thrash, M.D., medical director for the Uchee

Pines Institute in Seale, Alabama, sent this to me in 1988: "I have an experience for you. Early this year when I was on the West Coast, I saw a lady with a severe yeast problem—almost unable to eat anything, a lot of gas, bloating, discomfort, poor digestion, etc. She had tried everything, including Nystatin, with minimal help. I instructed her to take Japanese aged garlic extract in liquid form, three teaspoons three times a day, along with dietary changes and some other suggestions. She called me three months later to say that within two weeks her symptoms were all gone."

I spoke with Denning Cai, M.D., an Oriental physician specializing in family medicine in Hollywood, California, in 1991. She told me she has successfully used JAGE and various Chinese herbs in rebuilding the immune systems of many of her patients suffering from candida. She finds that the combination of aged garlic extract from Japan and medicinal plant extracts from China work better than when they are used independently.

A number of published reports appearing in the scientific literature of late demonstrates just how effective aged garlic extract can be for candida. Three of the best articles appeared in *Chemical and Pharmaceutical Bulletin* (36:3659–63, 1988), *Antimicrobial Agents and Chemotherapy* (30:499–501, Sept. 1986), and *International Clinical Nutrition Review* (10:423–29, Oct. 1990).

An interesting study, which appeared in the German scientific periodical *Zeitbibliothek der Bakterien und der Hygiene* (Journal of Bacteria and Hygiene) (I Abt. Orig. A 245: 229–39, 1979), showed that certain bacteria and yeast, including candida, become resistant to synthetic antibiotics over time, but they never acquire any resistance to compressed garlic juice.

What seem efficacious here are both the liquids (fluid extract and juice) and tablet/capsule versions of garlic. Up to 10 drops of the former and four to eight of the latter are recom-

mended. A garlic infusion or decoction, or a garlic liquer, vinegar, or wine, or just fresh garlic juice diluted in water, would
all make effective douches. A garlic bolus with a little live cultured yogurt added to it might be handy to use. (See pages 134
and 136 for information about how to make each of these.)

COMMON COLD AND INFLUENZA

Colds and flu rank as the most prevalent infectious
diseases around. In fact, the first chapter of my book *Double
the Power of Your Immune System* was devoted to them. My
very first recommendation is to get plenty of rest or vitamin
Zz *before* using garlic or any other health food supplements
or herbs. Most Americans, I've discovered over the years,
suffer from "sleep deprivation." There is no greater asset to
health than proper rest. An average of eight hours each day
is normal for most people, but if your body needs more,
then take it by all means!

Animals seem to have an innate sense of understanding
that garlic will do them good when they become sick. Consider this curious piece of news in the March 1961 issue of
Atlantic Monthly, which told of a flu epidemic striking Cape
Town, South Africa. Baboons who became sick with the respiratory disease were seen burrowing for wild garlic and
gorging themselves with it. Rural settlers sick with the flu
themselves, upon observing this strange behavior, started
hunting for it, too, and found considerable relief for their
raging fevers and congestions.

Just four years later, in 1965, a huge influenza epidemic
struck many parts of the Soviet Union. The Soviet government
flew in a *500 ton* emergency supply of raw garlic and the *Mos-
cow Evening News* encouraged citizens to eat more garlic because of its "prophylactic qualities for preventing flu."

Medical doctors with the common sense to use garlic

instead of antibiotics for treating flu cases have been amazed by the results. One German physician, J. Klosa, M.D., reported the success he had with a combination of garlic and onion in the March 1950 edition of *Medical Monthly*, a German periodical. He treated clogged and runny noses, sore throats, coughs, and other cold symptoms with two grams of garlic oil in a kilogram of water—plus some onion juice—20 to 25 drops every four hours. This treatment was taken by mouth and also in the nostrils.

He wrote that in all 31 cases of grippe (a severe, many-symptom cold), fever and catarrh were ended much quicker than by the usual treatment, with no lingering side effects. Also, considerable improvement was noticed in lung inflammation, swollen lymph glands, cough, jaundice, and pain in muscles and joints. Each of 28 cases of sore throat cleared up in 24 hours—more quickly if treated in the early stages. Seventy-one individuals with stuffy or runny noses got total relief in 13 to 20 minutes with no complications.

William H. Khoe, M.D., of Ojai, California, has also prescribed garlic for his patients instead of giving them flu shots. He recommends they take 10 capsules a day of JAGE in conjunction with 10 grams of vitamin C. He claims the garlic works better with ascorbic acid than without it. I've discovered in my own research that garlic is best taken just before retiring at night for *maximum* antibiotic effects. I've tested it on some of my students and office staff in times past, having those who've been sick with colds or flu take garlic in the daytime or at night. Invariably those who took it at night reported feeling better sooner than those who took the same amount in the daytime.

Even Jane E. Brody, health writer of *The New York Times*, recommended in one of her October 1984 columns plenty of raw garlic for any of her readers suffering with the sneezes and sniffles. She also wrote that its benefits may be preventive as well: "At the least, if you eat lots of garlic every day, it should keep people who carry cold viruses at enough of a distance to prevent you from catching their infections!"

Scientists have also discovered that garlic is very good for the flu. A Japanese researcher, K. Nagai, used JAGE to protect mice from infection with intranasally-inoculated influenza virus. The liquid extract was further shown to enhance the production of neutralizing antibody when given together with influenza vaccine (*Japanese Journal of Infectious Diseases* 47:321, 1973). Two Romanian virologists from Bucharest duplicated the same research with their own aqueous garlic extract administered intranasally or intramuscularly in mice infected with flu virus and achieved similar success (*Revue Roumaine De Medecine-Virologie* 34:11–17, 1983). And, finally, the Japanese science journal *Treatment and New Medicines* (22:1–22, December 1, 1985) reported the results of liquid JAGE administered to 39 patients suffering from common colds. Patients received one milliliter twice daily. Many of the symptoms such as headache, chill, chest abdominal and joint pains, fatigue, and lack of appetite noticeably improved following treatment.

Here is a simple plan for dealing with colds and flu. First, omit from the diet all red meat, sugary foods, dairy products, eggs, greasy foods, and soft drinks. Second, take plenty of water into the body, mostly quite warm. Third, get plenty of rest! And fourth, bombard the body with every type of garlic preparation you can think of! Declare all-out war on cold and flu germs until you've gained victory over them.

Soak in hot garlic baths often; these can be either full, half, or hand and foot baths. Drink plenty of garlic soup, broth, and tea. Apply a little garlic essence to the forehead, neck, and throat to relieve aches and pains. Apply hot garlic fomentations to the chest often. Take a dozen garlic capsules or tablets a day. Be sure to clean out the colon with a lukewarm but strong garlic enema. Rub some garlic liniment on the chest and inside the nostrils, if necessary, to faciliate breathing. Take some garlic liqueur, vinegar, and wine by the tablespoon to give you some pep and vitality. When you begin to feel better, enjoy a tossed salad made with romaine lettuce, endive, or spinach leaves (not iceberg lettuce), flavored with garlic oil and garlic vinegar. Use garlic oil to cook with, too. Gargle with garlic vinegar and a pinch of salt to relieve a sore throat. Another outstanding remedy that really works, though it burns for a moment, is to squeeze some drops of garlic juice towards the back of the throat followed immediately with 40 percent strength liquid bee propolis. It will feel as if you've just swallowed fire, but the sensation will pass in about a minute. If the cold or flu is prolonged, make a garlic-mustard plaster and put it on the chest overnight. Smoking handmade garlic cigarettes or burning garlic incense in the house will kill the cold or flu germs lingering in the air. Inserting a garlic suppository in the rectum at night just before going to bed is helpful. Calm a sore throat and nagging cough with teaspoon doses of garlic syrup taken throughout the day.

If you've managed to do most or all of this and get 12 to 15 hours sleep per day while you're sick, you'll be over it in no time at all, much to the amazement of your friends and family, who will probably still be struggling with their flu for days or even weeks to come.

CONTAGIOUS DISEASES

See pages 46-47 and 106-112.

CORNS AND CALLUSES

Benjamin Mamoud, M.D., a Cairo-based physician, provided me with this remedy for getting rid of corns and calluses on the soles of the feet when I was in Egypt in 1980. Cut slices of garlic to cover the part to be treated and fix them in place overnight with adhesive tape. Repeat this for several nights in succession and terminate the treatment with a cataplasm or paste of clay if the region being treated is irritated. In the case of warts or small cysts, it is at times preferable to rub the part affected with half a clove of garlic rather than to use a cataplasm, but in either case it's important that the treatment be finished with a cataplasm of clay.

CORONARY ARTERY DISEASE

This condition and atherosclerosis are the major killers in modern society. So wrote Dr. Benjamin Lau in the opening line of his chapter on garlic for the prevention of heart disease in the book *New Protective Roles for Selected Nutrients*. To differentiate between the two, think of coronary artery disease as an interruption of the normal flow of blood through the right and left coronary arteries of the heart, which can result in an atrophy or shrinkage of the heart muscle itself in due time. Atherosclerosis is the steady build-up of fatty plaque within these arteries, producing the slowdown in blood circulation. (See also "Arteriosclerosis and Atherosclerosis" for more details.)

Dr. Arun K. Bordia (cited earlier), a cardiologist from Udaipur, India, administered garlic oil capsules to patients suffering from coronary artery disease. He reported in the journal *Atherosclerosis* (28:155–59, 1977) that their ability to dissolve blood clots "increased under garlic feeding by

about 95 percent over that in the initial post-infarction period." He also noted that when garlic was taken with a high-
fat meal, it not only prevented a drop in the body's ability
to dissolve blood clots, it also increased this action beyond
the normal rate by almost 15 percent within the third hour.
"This shows that garlic acts within a few hours," he observed.

The Department of Public Information at Pennsylvania
State University sent out a press release dated August 29,
1990, under the heading "Garlic May Help Reduce Heart
Disease Risk." It quoted Dr. Yu-Yan Yeh, an associate professor of nutrition in Penn State's College of Health and
Human Development, as saying that garlic seems to lower
excess blood fats, including cholesterol and triglycerides,
which circulate in the body. Yeh had added Japanese aged
garlic extract to the diet of laboratory rats in an effort to
determine how effectively this was carried out. "In such animal studies," he said, "we have found that a diet of which
two percent was garlic is effective in lowering plasma cholesterol and triglyceride levels." High elevations of both are
one of the primary causes of coronary artery disease.

At the World Garlic Congress in 1990, additional information corroborating Yeh's findings was presented by scientists from the University of Wisconsin and the University of
Limburg in The Netherlands. Garlic capsules, tablets, liqueur, oil, vinegar, and wine should be used frequently
along with raw garlic to prevent this disease.

CUTS

Garlic can effectively replace Mercurochrome or tincture of iodine in treating minor cuts, but it must be used
judiciously, since it can irritate the skin. Garlic juice, tea,
fluid extract, liniment, liqueur, ointment, packing, powder,

fomentation, hot vinegar compress, and wine bath are all useful for preventing infection.

DIABETES

Attention diabetics! If you want an herb that will really help bring down your elevated blood sugar levels and may even reduce your insulin dependency, then *raw* garlic and American and European manufactured brands of garlic are the things for you. A German physician, Dr. Madaus, reported in the journal *Lehrbuch der Biologischen Heilmittel* (Textbook of Biological Remedies) (1:479) that garlic can reduce the blood sugar in some cases of diabetes mellitus. He described a patient taking 100 cc of insulin daily with sugar in the urine of eight percent, and a blood sugar count of 242 mg. After the patient started taking EMG capsules (three twice a day) for one week, he only registered two percent urinary sugar and 215 mg. of blood sugar.

However, what works well for one may be detrimental to others. People who have hypoglycemia may want to rethink their use of raw garlic and American and European garlic preparations. Four separately published studies definitely show that garlic in these forms may cause hypoglycemic reactions: *The Lancet* (2:1491, 1973); *The American Journal of Clinical Nutrition* (28:684, July 1975); *Medikon* (6:15–18, 1977); and *Journal of Ethnobotany* (15:121–32, February 1986). However, in conversation with Dr. Benjamin Lau in 1990, I learned that Japanese aged garlic extracts are quite safe for those with low blood sugar and will not induce hypoglycemic reactions such as sudden fatigue, forgetfullness, mood swings, and insomnia.

In addition to garlic, cayenne pepper, goldenseal root, and pau d'arco are decidedly hypoglycemic and while of definite benefit to diabetics, they are not recommended for those with low blood sugar problems.

Raw garlic, garlic juice, capsules, tablets, liqueur, tea or soup, vinegar, and wine are the best forms for diabetics to use.

DIARRHEA AND DYSENTERY

If you're going to a Third World country where the food and water may be suspect, be sure to take along an ample supply of garlic capsules, tablets, or fluid extract. They will come in handy and help to check any diarrhea you may pick up on your trip.

For E. E. Marcovici, M.D., his experiences with garlic began in the trenches of World War I, where he was in charge of experimental studies on preventing and curing gastrointestinal infections like diarrhea. Writing in the *Medical Record* (153:63–65, 1941) a quarter of a century later, he described how giving an entire garlic bulb a day to dysentery patients produced a rapid subjective and objective return to health, often within less than a week. Later on he used a preparation made by the Sandoz Pharmaceutical Company, in which garlic was absorbed into charcoal and slowly released as it passed along the digestive tract. After the war, Marcovici conducted further experiments to verify his wartime experiences. He gave 2.5 grams of garlic powder to patients and found that this completely protected them from a dose of dysenteric organisms that would otherwise have killed them ten times over.

Doctors F. Damrau and E. A. Ferguson reviewed 29 successful cures of diarrhea and other stomach complaints with the use of garlic in the *Review of Gastroenterology* (16:411–19, 1949). They cited the case of a 55-year-old woman who had, for an entire year, experienced a series of gastrointestinal problems, including diarrhea, belching, gas, and appetite loss. She was given two tablets of dehydrated garlic twice daily after meals and, within two weeks, the symptoms were nearly gone.

A Phoenix physician I know, who regularly treats diarrhea in young children due to celiac disease (gluten intolerance), says that garlic is the best remedy he knows of. He routinely uses EMG from Germany for this problem, finding it works better than the American brands he has tried.

Since unfriendly bacteria are known to cause diarrhea, this next piece of research may confirm garlic's usefulness in the diet to prevent loose stool. Indian researchers reported in the *Journal of Scientific and Industrial Research* (16C:173–74, 1957) of feeding four rats a stock diet which included 2.5 percent garlic for five days. Feces samples were collected on the last two days. Two species of gram-negative bacteria, Escherichia aurescens and E. coli, and several species of another gram-negative bacteria belonging to the genus Bacteroides—all of which occur in the colon—were greatly reduced by the presence of garlic.

EARACHE

Eleonore Blaurock-Busch, who wrote an herb column entitled "Eleonore's Herbals" for *Bestways* health magazine for many years, interviewed me some years ago for one of her articles. Somehow we got on the subject of garlic and earaches and she told me, "During her preschool years, my daughter Yvette developed an ear infection. Like any concerned parent, I took her to a medical specialist, who confirmed the diagnosis. He also noticed a rupture of the eardrum. After his extensive examination, we were given a prescription for an antibiotic, which was to be taken for 10 days. Although I am extremely fond of this doctor, the thought of treating a minor ear infection with powerful anti-biotics did not appeal to me one bit.

"I remembered my grandmother's remedies and went to work. Yvette had to swallow two garlic oil capsules four times daily for the first three days, after which the dose was reduced to a total of six capsules daily. I applied warm chamomile and potato poultices and had her take vitamins A, B, C, and the mineral calcium. Within two days, the pain and discomfort were gone. Her health rapidly improved after that.

"After two weeks, we went for our scheduled medical appointment, and the specialist was pleased with her progress. There was no more sign of an infection, and the eardrum had healed. My daughter is now 13 years old and never had to take any synthetic antibiotics."

Hsu Wei-cheng, M.D., a researcher with the Ear, Nose, and Throat Department of the Inner Mongolia Medical College in Huhehot, reported in the *Chinese Medical Journal* (3:204–5, May 1977) of having used tissue-thin slices of fresh garlic in repairing eardrum perforations in 18 separate cases. The time required for healing by this method occupied the better part of two weeks in a dozen of the cases and almost a month in six other cases where the perforations were larger than half of the eardrum pars tensa. Ten to 19 decibels hearing was gained after therapy was completed. (NOTE: It is *not* recommended that this be attempted at home, since it was done by skilled surgeons in a hospital setting.)

Lukewarm garlic oil, tincture, or fluid extract would be useful for treating ear infections at home.

ECZEMA

Lillian T. Elders of St. Louis, Missouri related this to me in 1978: "For years I have been getting outbreaks of dry eczema on my toes and around my toenails. The itching was maddening at night when my feet got warm under the covers. I tried many remedies to no avail. Knowing the wonders of garlic, I decided to try that. I scraped some fresh cloves with a paring knife to get the oil loose and smeared the fiber and oil on my toes, rubbing it in well. I was amazed—no more itching—and the eczema healed." (NOTE: Some people have hypersensitive skin and this remedy may cause severe discomfort for them. It is advisable to first test it on a very tiny portion of the skin before using it over a larger area to see if any serious reactions occur.)

A garlic hand or foot bath may be efficacious for eczema, as well as a cold garlic compress or cold extract. A fomentation gently laid on top of the afflicted area may bring additional relief. A garlic liniment or ointment may be helpful, too. Garlic preparations made with alcohol are not recommended in this case.

FATIGUE

See the brief report from the Japanese journal *Treatment and New Medicines* cited under Common Cold and Influenza (page 86), for the strengthening benefits of JAGE on older patients weakened by respiratory ailments. Capsules of Japanese garlic extract (two daily), garlic essence, fluid extract, liqueur, vinegar, and wine will all act as tonics for revitalizing weakened bodies.

FOOD POISONING

A Catholic bishop, Monsignor David Greenstock, wrote an article in a Spanish language agricultural journal called *Ceres*, in which he made a strong case for using garlic as an effective agent to counteract the terribly painful effects of food poisoning.

In late December 1992 one of the worst outbreaks of infectious hepatitis occurred in Denver, Colorado. A large catering business, which had served food to 12,000 people at various corporate holiday parties, was shut down after state inspectors discovered contaminated food. The source of the hepatitis was traced to a number of temporary workers, hired through the holidays, who had used the restrooms but failed to wash their hands thoroughly afterwards.

Henry Champ, who works for a large computer firm in the area, told me by phone that a number of his fellow co-workers "got sicker than dogs, but neither my wife nor I felt as much as a burp" from the contaminated food they ate. "We're both crazy about garlic," he admitted. "Just can't seem to get enough of the stuff. Fact is, we fairly reek of it. My wife uses it about every day in whatever she cooks for supper. And I like to put raw slices of it on the sandwiches I take to work with me. I think this is what saved us from becoming sick in a big-time way."

Chu-Yen Luke, who runs an Oriental grocery store and teaches Chinese cooking in the evenings in Chicago, told me at a recent health convention held there, that he always uses garlic whenever he cooks a pork dish. "I do this because the pigs are not clean," he said. "They run around and eat everything, and they have all sorts of filth around them. The garlic kills the bad bugs they carry. For this same reason, I use garlic whenever there are swamp vegetables in a dish. It is used in everything I can think of except beef dishes."

Aflatoxins are naturally occurring and dangerous metabolites produced by *Aspergillus flavus* and related fungal species. Of the 16 or more toxic compounds secreted by these fungi, aflatoxin B-1 (AFB-1) exhibits the most potent biologic activity, causing cell mutations in various microorganisms as well as in animal and human cells, mutations that can eventually lead to cancer. It has also been linked to increased incidences of human liver cancer in Africa and Asia. It is of considerable concern that many food items consumed in the world, including peanuts, rice, grains, corn, beans, and sweet potatoes, are usually contaminated with AFB-1.

Drs. Benjamin Lau, Padma P. Tadi, and Robert W. Teel reported in *Nutrition and Cancer* journal (15:87–95, 1991) that isolated components of raw garlic, notably ajoene and diallyl sulfide, and JAGE prevented AFB-1 from binding to cell DNA matter, which ultimately neutralized this particularly toxic metabolite. They found that the liquid Japanese aged garlic extract did a better job of this than did two single garlic compounds.

The following garlic preparations are quite serviceable in treating food poisoning symptoms; they are listed according to their active potency for this problem: Japanese aged garlic extract liquid (two tablespoons) or in capsules (14 at a time), garlic infusion (two cups at one time), garlic fluid extract (45 drops), garlic syrup (two tablespoons), and garlic wine (three fluid ounces).

FREE RADICALS

For those still unfamiliar with free radicals, think of them as menacing sharks zipping around in your cellular sea. Better yet, they are molecules that carry an extra or unpaired electron. When you have one that isn't paired, it becomes highly reactive to the more complete and orderly molecules surrounding it. Sometimes that's good. For instance, free radicals are an important part of normal physiological processes such as digestion: free radicals help tear food apart and assist in converting it to energy. Free radicals are also used by the immune system as chemical "weapons" to attack bacterial and viral invaders. But more often than not, things tend to get out of hand with them. These wildly misbehaving "criminal" molecules can generate excessive oxygen and damage surrounding tissues, resulting in diseases like atherosclerosis, cancer, cataracts, Parkinson's, rheumatoid arthritis, and senility.

Garlic and onion are two of the very best spices to check the errant behavior of these free radicals. The late sociologist Belle Boone Beard studied 8,500 centenarians in her lifetime and discovered one common thread that ran throughout her huge survey. In profiling the eating habits of centenarians, two foods stood out above everything else: garlic and onion (*Science* 206:1057, November 30, 1979).

John C. Hansen of McKinleyville, California, who is well into his eighties, attributes his longevity to garlic. This is what he wrote to me in 1992: "Garlic has been one of my favorite foods and I am sure that it has had a lot to do with my age. . . . I used to try to get one of my brothers to take a little garlic. And he said there is no such thing as a little garlic. Another brother would never eat garlic or onions; said they stank too much. Well, both of my brothers have long left for realms unknown, but I'm still around because of my garlic. I soak some raw cloves in apple cider vinegar for 20 months. I shake the mixture up every day and keep adding some more vinegar as it evaporates. This is how I make my own aged garlic extract. Then I strain the stuff and take a big heaping tablespoonful every morning. I call it my 'tonic of life.' "

David Kritchevsky, associate director of Philadelphia's prestigious Wistar Institute and one of the first to explore garlic's cholesterol-lowering properties, told me the following story at the World Garlic Congress. There was a woman, he said, who admitted to being 66, but looked 44, and acted as if she were only 22. She attributed her vigor to the garlic clove in her nightly salad. Dr. Kritchevsky described her health program to his father, who quipped, "No wonder— the angel of death can't even get near her!"

At the World Garlic Congress, Dr. Robert I. Lin, the conference organizer, reported that Japanese aged garlic extract can protect isolated human hemoglobin and human red blood cells from oxidation and free radicals. On the other hand, he noted, raw garlic and products containing dried raw garlic powders can cause damage to hemoglobin and the red blood cells under similar conditions. He presented additional evidence to support his findings.

To help curb free radical activity, use garlic often. But based on some of the toxicological evidence which scientists have come up with lately, it may be a good idea to limit your use of raw garlic to meal preparation and instead use garlic medicinally in some other form. The most practical ones would be a garlic electuary, essence, fluid extract, capsule, liqueur, tablet, tincture, vinegar, or wine. Suggested amounts are given under each of these in the following chapter.

It is also best to take garlic preparations when eating fried, deep-fried, charbroiled, and refrigerated foods. Since all are high in free radicals to begin with, the ample use of garlic supplements will help to curtail their mischievous activities.

FUNGUS

More specific information on garlic's value in treating fungal yeast infection may be found under Candida in this chapter. But the following case history amply illustrates the importance of garlic therapy in fungal infection. This report first appeared in the January 1983 issue of the *Indian Journal of Dermatology* and has been reprinted with the kind permission of the authors and the journal.

Sporotrichosis from India has mostly been reported from the Northeastern region. . . . A young soldier aged 30 years, posted for some time in the Assam region, reported to us with a warty lesion on the ring finger of his left hand and six ulcers on the left forearm and arm of eight months duration. . . . The clinical picture was suggestive of sporotrichosis and our patient was investigated accordingly. . . .

While the fungus culture results were awaited, the patient was treated with a broad spectrum of antibiotics and local dressings with no visible improvement. Based on the in vitro sensitivity studies it was decided to study the effect of garlic juice on the lesions of the patient. . . . On the first day a garlic juice-soaked gauze was applied on the largest ulcer and kept in position with a light bandage.

An irritant reaction was noticed within 24 hours which made the ulcer look more angry and, therefore, a second application was not done. The ulcer was kept covered with dry sterile gauze. Within 3 days, however, the ulcer showed remarkable improvement. A second application done after 4 days produced mild irritation again. The ulcer healed completely within ten days. Due to the satisfactory results, the garlic juice was applied on the remaining lesions similarly and kept in position for 24 hours. The patient tolerated the mild irritation well. No second application was required on most of the lesions, which healed over a period of 6–13 days after a single application. The patient was kept in the hospital for 2 weeks to see if there was any recurrence. He was reviewed again after 6 weeks, 3 months, and 6 months with no evidence of recurrence being noticed.

The best garlic preparations for treating a condition such as this, whether it be on the upper arm, forearm, hand, or between the fingers, toes, or groin area are as follows: cold extract, gauze soaked in fluid extract, fomentation, fresh garlic juice, liniment, garlic oil, an ointment, a poultice or plaster, or gauze soaked in garlic vinegar.

When putting any of these applications on the infected area, be sure to watch carefully for any undue reactions. If the area becomes too highly inflamed, discontinue treatment at once and see a dermatologist.

HEART ATTACKS

Science News (138:157) for September 8, 1988, reported on an interesting study involving garlic to prevent heart attacks. Four hundred thirty-two heart attack survivors were equally divided into two groups. Half of the participants consumed the juice from six to ten cloves of fresh garlic a day. The other half took a garlic-scented placebo. Overall, the garlic eaters suffered 32 percent fewer recurrent heart attacks and 45 percent fewer deaths from heart attacks than the unsupplemented patients.

In August, 1987 the Mayor of New York City, Ed Koch, suffered a mild stroke. Dr. J. P. Mohr, head of the Stroke Center at Columbia-Presbyterian Medical Center, prescribed a daily aspirin for hizzoner and also put him on a strict low-fat, low-salt diet with lots of fresh fruits and vegetables. Koch was permitted to keep eating a modified form of Chinese cuisine, particularly dishes with an edible fungus called moer, or tree ear mushrooms. Dr. Mohr also recommended Chinese dishes with garlic. Both of these, he told a press conference, were marvelous bloodthinners to keep his patient, the Mayor, from getting another heart attack.

A garlic decoction, electuary, essence, fluid extraction, gelatin capsules, infusion, liqueur, oil, pill, syrup, tablet, tincture, vinegar, and wine are all good to use in stroke prevention. But the one I like best is my own recipe which I call Green Garlic Elixir:

> In a medium saucepan, combine one large head of garlic, separated into cloves and peeled, with two cups of chicken or vegetable broth. Boil, then reduce to simmer for 15 minutes. Put the mixture with two bunches of parsley into a blender and puree. Season with kelp and drink daily.

HEAVY METAL POISONING

Both *Runner's World* and *Omni* magazines for May 1979 reported on experiments in Japan and the Soviet Union that showed the pungent cloves of garlic absorb lead, mercury, cadmium, and other toxic metals in the body, which then can be excreted during bowel movements. Both publications reminded city joggers who breathe the exhaust fumes of traffic while exercising that they should remember to take garlic each day to remain healthy.

The Japanese study conducted by Drs. Ikezoe and Kitahara used Japanese aged garlic extract. They conducted controlled studies on rabbits and humans. The method of study was: observation of the release of potassium and hemoglobin by heavy metals from erythrocytes, and destruction of erythrocyte membrane. Their conclusion was that JAGE prevented the poisoning effect from heavy metals and protected the erythrocyte membrane from destruction.

Dr. Benjamin Lau of Loma Linda University School of Medicine conducted an even simpler experiment to demonstrate the role of garlic in preventing heavy metal poisoning. Ten test tubes were each set up with 15 milliliters of a five percent suspension of human red blood cells. In the first tube was added a 0.5 milliliter saline solution and in the second tube was added 0.5 milliliter of a one to ten dilution of liquid Japanese aged garlic extract. Other tubes had heavy metals, such as lead acetate, mercury, copper, and aluminum added to give a final concentration of 500 µM. For each pair of tubes with heavy metal salts, one received the saline solution and the other a diluted JAGE solution. In every instance the heavy metal salts caused the red blood cells to undergo destruction, but the presence of small quantities of JAGE solution prevented this destruction of red blood cells in some test tubes (*International Clinical Nutrition Review* 9:27–28, January 1989).

The best forms of garlic for prevention in this case would be raw garlic used in cooking, raw garlic juice in some type of liquid chlorophyll drink, garlic oil capsules, and a good garlic broth or tea.

HEMORRHOIDS

Dr. LeRoy Fitzsimmons of Bath, England, recommends this remedy to his patients suffering from piles. They are instructed to bathe the area with warm water and mild soap, after which they apply either garlic juice or diluted crushed garlic with absorbent cotton three to five times. He also recommends a sitzbath of warm water containing the juice squeezed from four garlic cloves. The patient should sit in this for 10 minutes.

Another method is to apply cold garlic compresses morning and evening to the rectum. Then some white petroleum jelly should be rubbed inside the rectal area, after which thin slices of a peeled clove should be carefully inserted and left overnight.

George Barany, a chemist and garlic researcher at the University of Minnesota, is fond of telling this tale. Several years ago at an elegant dinner, he introduced himself to the woman on his right. Later, between courses, his neighbor leaned over, smiled, and explained how she had banished her hemorrhoids by inserting whole garlic cloves as suppositories. "It's absolutely unbelievable what people are apt to tell me over filet mignon or prime rib," he confessed.

HIVES

Doris Heinz, a registered nurse from Grandview, Washington, wrote to me some time ago to mention that rubbing a cut clove of garlic over hives reduces the itching. "It soothes and soon they are forgotten or the blisters start to heal," she said. This may work well, but readers are again reminded that not every person's skin will respond so kindly to something as strong as garlic, especially when there is already an outbreak on the surface. This should be tried on a small area first, just to make sure there is no untoward reaction.

A garlic cold compress, cold extract, decoction rinse, fomentation, juice, liniment, ointment, and poultice would be good for hives, too.

HYPERCHOLESTEROLEMIA

This is a fancy medical term to indicate an abnormally large amount of cholesterol in the cells and plasma of the circulating blood. Garlic is capable of reversing this, but with some surprises that astonished researchers.

Dr. Benjamin Lau of Loma Linda University Medical School started his first experiment using Japanese aged garlic extract with 32 volunteers suffering from hypercholesterolemia. He naturally expected to see a reduction of their cholesterol levels, so imagine his surprise when just the reverse happened. The Japanese aged garlic extract he and his

team used actually increased the test subjects' serum cholesterol and triglycerides in the first two months!

"We were ready to abandon our research," he said,
"until we found out from other researchers using only raw
garlic that the same thing had happened with their patients,
too." Dr. Lau postulated that garlic moves lipids from their
storage place in the tissues and deposits them into the bloodstream. United States Department of Agriculture researchers
discovered the same thing: rats fed garlic extract for 18 days
had a few lipid deposits in the liver but much higher lipids
in their circulating blood plasma.

Dr. Lau's outlook brightened as the experiment moved
into its third month. "We saw a significant drop in the
serum lipids of our volunteers who took JAGE," he reported. "They reached a low level in six months." His expla-
nation for all of this? "We believe, based on our research,
that garlic causes lipid deposits to shift into the bloodstream,
causing higher blood lipid levels at first, but later, with continued garlic intake, excess serum lipids are broken down
and passed off through the intestinal tract. Several other
non-related studies have reported that this actually occurs
in animals who are fed garlic."

The work of Drs. Suzanne G. Yu and A. A. Qureshi is
of interest here, too. They supplemented corn-based diets
normally fed to hypercholesterolemic chickens with either
garlic powder (4 percent), garlic oil (0.03 percent), various
doses of JAGE (0.3 to 8.1 percent), or S-allyl-cysteine (15
ppm to 405 ppm), an important sulphur component of garlic. At the 1991 National Conference on Cholesterol and
High Blood Pressure in Washington, D.C., where this research was presented, they reported that the Japanese aged
garlic extract and S-allyl-cysteine strongly inhibited further
rise in serum cholesterol in these chickens. The other two
garlic preparations did not perform as well.

A study carried out at John Bastyr College of Naturopathic Medicine in Seattle, Washington, a few years ago suggests that garlic oil may still help prevent the onset of heart disease. In a rigorous investigation into the therapeutic properties of garlic, researchers found that 20 healthy student volunteers who ate 18 mg. of encapsulated garlic oil a day for four weeks enjoyed significantly higher levels of beneficial (HDL) cholesterol, lower blood pressure, and less blood clotting than when the same subjects ate placebo capsules for two weeks (*Journal of Orthomolecular Medicine* 2:15–21, 1987).

Further evidence from a German study of just a few years ago indicates that garlic in tablet form may lower total cholesterol levels. Two hundred sixty-one patients who had total cholesterol levels higher than 200 mg/dl were given either European manufactured garlic in 800 mg. amounts or a placebo for four months. Those given the EMG tablets had a mean 12 percent and 17 percent reduction in serum cholesterol and triglyceride levels (*Medical Tribune* 32 (10):4).

For reducing very severe hypercholesterolemia, the combination of garlic and guar gum seem to work best. A recent study in Finland demonstrated the effectiveness of guar gum in the treatment of very high hypercholesterolemia. Fifteen to thirty grams of guar gum per day reduced serum cholesterol 12 to 20 percent in patients (*Atherosclerosis* 72:157–62, 1988). Garlic capsules or tablets (four daily) in conjunction with capsules of guar gum (three daily) is recommended. Also, any of the other garlic preparations mentioned in the next chapter, which are alcohol-based, would be helpful, as would raw garlic itself.

HYPERTENSION

High blood pressure responds well to garlic. Here are two patients' experiences.

Hugh L. Hill of Washington, Indiana wrote to me in 1979 to report, "In April, 1975, I was directed by a railroad M.D. to start taking a drug for my blood pressure as it was 156/90. I was to report back to him in three weeks. Meanwhile I went to see my own doctor, as I had problems breathing while taking the drug. He put me on another medication for hypertension. Then someone told me I ought to try garlic. So I started taking garlic capsules along with the medication. My blood pressure came down to about 130/72 by taking five capsules of garlic a day. In February, 1977, my blood pressure was down to 110/76, so I discontinued my medication and just stayed with the garlic after that."

Mrs. Ilene Hastings of White Cliffs, New York, wrote me the following in 1975: "A 36-year-old, heavy-set friend of mine was plagued by high blood pressure. She had tried various prescribed medications with only limited success and often undesirable side affects. Then on a visit to her family home in Alabama, a wise old aunt suggested she try taking some chopped garlic in a tablespoon of apple cider vinegar each morning. After some understandable initial skepticism, my friend awoke one morning and began a daily regimen of this new 'medicine.' Within a few weeks, she felt much better and her lifelong high blood pressure was slowly receding. A visit to her physician confirmed this and he was apparently as delighted as she was."

Any of the garlic preparations mentioned in Chapter 6 intended for internal consumption will be useful for reducing hypertension, but garlic capsules, tablets, oil, fluid extract, vinegar, and wine seem to be the most effective.

INFECTIOUS DISEASES

The clinical literature shows that garlic is suited for even the very worst types of infections. During World War I

British medics wrapped gangrenous wounds in garlic-soaked bandages and saved many an infected limb from amputation.

Leprosy, or Hansen's disease, is induced by an organism very similar to the one that causes tuberculosis and is exceptionally difficult to treat. However, in India, which has many of the world's cases of this disease, garlic has been successfully used to combat it when all other forms of conventional therapy have failed. The *Journal of the Indian Medical Association* (39:517–21, 1962) presented evidence and case studies to support this fact.

A deadly form of meningitis occurs when the meninges—the membranes enclosing the brain and spinal cord—become infected by a yeastlike fungus known as *Cryptococcus neoformans*. Many untreated patients die within months, but conventional therapy with amphotericin B has cut mortality to about 15 percent. However, the drug is not without severe side effects, such as permanent kidney damage, convulsions, and generalized pain.

The Chinese Medical Journal (93:123, Feb. 1980) reported that after a garlic extract was given orally plus either intramuscularly or intravenously over a period of several weeks to 21 patients suffering from *Cryptococcal meningitis*, 11 experienced noticeable improvement. Of these, six were totally cured; all their symptoms had vanished and fungi could no longer be found in their cerebrospinal fluid. Five other cases improved dramatically, while the remaining five died. Of the five who were given conventional drugs, two were cured, two improved slightly, and one died. Doctors concluded that garlic is the best therapy for reduction of the transient chills, low-grade fever, headache, nausea, vomiting, and pain accompanying this disease.

In 1979 when I went to the Soviet Union with a group of other scientists, we met with a physician in Leningrad

who showed us clinical studies on the positive effects of
raw garlic extract for the successful management of multiple
sclerosis. He also produced a number of his own patients'
records, which detailed the favorable improvement of their
conditions while on his garlic therapy program. One of my
colleagues, the late Dr. Walter McKain, who understood
Russian a lot better than I did, gave a verbal translation of
the more significant data for my benefit.

The most efficacious preparation of garlic this Russian
physician had found was a fluid extract. He made it by
grinding 350 grams of garlic and mixing it with 200 milliliters of Russian vodka. This he set in a dark place for ten
days, shaking five times daily. Then he filtered it three times.
He would start his patients on one drop the first morning
in milk, two drops the second morning, three drops the
third, and so forth until they had reached 25 drops on the
25th day. Upon reaching this peak, they continued taking
25 drops every day in milk until completely cured. He testi-
fied to having achieved a 59 percent cure rate.

Virologists working out of the University of Michigan
reported in *Antibiotics Annual 1958–1959* (pp. 104–109) that
a fluid extract combination of elephant garlic and St. Johnswort reduced the incidence of poliomyelitis in mice to
under 64 percent.

The following item, a reader's report of her tuberculosis
cure, appeared in the *Vegetarian News Digest* for September–October, 1949:

> I had been confined in a Western hospital for about
> seven years with T.B. ... A new nurse appeared. ...
> After the nurse heard my problem ... she said, "When
> you arrive home get about two pounds of garlic into the
> house and keep plenty of it on hand. Take one ounce of
> peeled garlic daily, preferably between meals, chop it
> finely and crush and eat it in a cupful of soup, in carrot

juice or other vegetable juice; in any way which you take it, do so gradually until at the end of the week you will be eating three to four ounces daily; by then the poisons will start eliminating from the body so that you will think you will die—but you won't. . . . During the purgation period it is well to assist the cleansing process by drinking all the liquids possible, between meals (no coffee or tea at any time); vegetable and fruit juices, being careful not to mix them, are recommended. . . . Take garlic enemas after each bowel movement. . . .

"You can put finely chopped garlic on a piece of paper and, while resting, inhale its odor for minutes at a time. No matter how people may ostracize you, just continue using it. . . . In about three months time you will . . . grow strong enough in a short time to lead a normal life."

. . . I followed the nurse's instruction to the letter, and, as my husband did not object, I ate garlic in every way I could think of—with green string beans, diced carrots, etc. I would cut up a clove of garlic and add it to the boiling liquid two to three minutes before turning off the fire, then add two spoonfuls of soy or olive oil and eat it with the liquid. I prepared cream cheese with chopped celery or parsley leaves and then mixed garlic with some. I, of course, crushed it and mixed it with French dressing and used it over all vegetable salads.

During the purgative period my body eliminated such black mucus and "sick" liquid, I hardly could believe it was inside me. With the aid of fruit and vegetable juices and daily enemas, after about four weeks' time my bowel excrement became normal and life seemed worth living again.

When I went to the hospital for a checkup, the orthodox doctors did not recognize me; neither would they believe me when I told them about "the cure." One remarked that "nothing like that had ever been used before, etc., etc." X-rays, however, do not lie and they gave me a clean bill of health, despite their total disbelief.

Early in this century Dr. William Minchin found himself in charge of the TB ward of the Kells Union Hospital in Dublin, Ireland. One day an 18-year-old boy with severe tuberculosis of the right leg and foot refused the amputation Minchin suggested. Six months later he saw the boy in his home town walking without much difficulty.

Dr. Minchin asked him how this miracle occurred. The boy told of going to see a farmer named Charles Walker of County Meath, who was famous for having a secret remedy for TB in his family, which consisted of a poultice containing soot, salt, and powdered garlic. By trial and error experimentation, Dr. Minchin eventually learned that the garlic was the only active ingredient. This he began to use in his own hospital treatments. He applied garlic oil externally on the infected part, gave large amounts of the raw clove in the diet and, for TB of the lungs, his patients were instructed to inhale the oil vapors for one hour three times a day through a specially-made inhalant device.

He found he could successfully treat almost every case that came to him, provided there was some kind of passage of air to and from the tubercular area of the lungs. He compiled a book of the more interesting cases cured with garlic and included his correspondence with other doctors who had adopted his therapy for their patients as well. The book, *The Treatment of Tuberculosis with Oleum Allii* (garlic oil), was published in 1915.

Nearly three-quarters of a century later, Edward Delaha and Vincent F. Garagusi of Georgetown University Hospital set out to confirm the work of Dr. Minchin. They added a European manufactured garlic extract to 30 strains of mycobacteria growing in test tubes. A month later, the garlic had done critical damage to all 30 strains. Garagusi said that they were both astounded at what happened.

It is said on good authority by some of his biographers, that the great scientist-physician-philosopher Albert Schweitzer used garlic to treat cases of typhus and cholera.

A British doctor of some renown addressed a London conference of physicians at the Royal Medical Society some years ago. He told this august body that he had just learned something from an old peasant woman that made him feel both glad and idiotic.

He said that all of the attempts he and his distinguished colleagues had made in treating whooping cough in children had virtually failed. But a simple home remedy taught to him by this unschooled but very wise woman had never failed to work on even the most stubborn case of whooping cough. She had used it for over half a century, he said, and had never once lost a child.

With obvious regret, he admitted that no one in the meeting hall could make such a claim. In fact, he had lost more than his share of youngsters because the standard remedies of the day did them more harm than good. But, he reported, in the short time he had been using this old woman's remedy, he had not lost a single patient.

Her remedy was garlic, and it was used in the form of a poultice on the soles of the feet. First, you remove the outer peels from the small sections of cloves and chop them up fine enough to make a poultice about a quarter of an inch thick to cover the bottom of each foot. Next, spread it evenly on a piece of soft muslin cloth and place a thin piece of cloth over the garlic, remembering to grease the bottoms of the feet with hog lard or petroleum jelly. If the garlic is placed directly on the feet without the benefit of some type of lubricant, it's apt to burn and blister. Now place the prepared poultice on a cloth suitable for binding it overnight.

It is wise to cover the foot and poultice with an old sock so the poultice will not be kicked off during the night. Remove it carefully in the morning, as the same poultice may be used several times. After that, make a fresh one and proceed as before. You will smell garlic on the patient's breath the morning after each application. This same treatment, he concluded, will work quite satisfactorily in the case of anyone having a hard night's cough. This appeared in the British health publication *Nature's Path* in June, 1945.

Mary T. Quelch, a British herbalist, recommended in her book *Herbs For Daily Use* that wafer-thin slices of garlic be laid around in the bottom of a large soup bowl. Over them pour just enough maple syrup or blackstrap molasses to cover and let it stand for five hours. By that time the syrup or molasses and the juice of the garlic will have sufficiently mixed. A person troubled by whooping cough, smoker's cough, asthma, or bronchitis should then take one teaspoon several times a day, as needed.

Just about all of the garlic preparations mentioned in Chapter Six will be useful here for any type of infectious disease. However, it appears that the less processing done to raw garlic, the more potent it will be. In other words, manufactured brands of garlic will be of some benefit, but they are usually not as effective as straight, raw garlic.

INSECT PROBLEMS

Garlic is one of the best natural insect repellants I know of. The following material, which has been accumulated over a couple of decades, supports this.

From Ruth Haigner of Pittsburgh, Pennsylvania: "Grind up some cloves of garlic and add them to your manure tea barrel and rain barrel to prevent mosquitoes from breeding in them. I had this problem one year, even with a lid on the barrel, but after I used the garlic, no more mosquito larvae. It's good to spray on plants for killing aphids, worms, and bugs, too."

From Geraldine Klompers of San Jose, California: "I'd like to share my experience with you in keeping fleas off my little pet poodle named Killer. I had almost lost her from using so many different kinds of commercial flea sprays. So I began to think about fleas being similar to fruit tree pests. My husband and I keep some citrus and olive trees in our backyard. We always plant garlic around them to keep pests away. So I started giving Killer one garlic capsule every other day. I would mix it in with her regular chow. It's been five months now and she hasn't had a flea since. Her coat is beautiful beyond description. Bigger dogs might need two capsules a day."

Millie Roper of Reedley, California, attended a senior citizen horticulture class in the Spring of 1987 and learned how to make an excellent, all-purpose insecticide. "We soaked lots of finely minced raw garlic in mineral oil for at least 24 hours. About two teaspoons of this oil was then added to a pint of tap water in which one-fourth ounce of dish detergent had been dissolved. This was thoroughly stirred, then strained into a glass container for storage. When used as a spray, one to two tablespoons of oil was blended into a pint of water."

She claimed that this garlic insecticide worked on cabbage moths and loopers, earwigs, leafhoppers, mosquitoes (including their larvae), whiteflies, aphids, houseflies, June, squash, and lygus bugs, cockroaches, slugs, and hornworms. Some were killed immediately on contact, while the rest took several minutes to kill. Ladybugs, Colorado potato beetles, grasshoppers, grape leaf skeletonizers, red ants, and sow bugs were not affected.

If you want to keep insect pests away while out hiking

in nature, try squeezing a garlic perle into some petroleum jelly and rub it on your arms, face and neck. Taking some of the garlic internally will afford you double protection.

If bitten or stung by an insect, hastily chew a raw garlic clove and apply the saliva mixture to the injured site. Carefully remove the stinger first. It will give prompt relief!

Two entomologists from the University of California proved in 1972 that garlic is an effective insecticide. Using what they called a "crude extract of garlic," Drs. Elden L. Reeves and Sankar V. Amonkar discovered that it caused 100 percent mortality in five different species of mosquito larvae when used in such small doses as 200 parts per million (ppm). They used a crude methanolic extract of commercially available dehydrated garlic, called instant minced garlic, and also a more refined form obtained from freshly reconstituted dehydrated garlic by steam distillation. Both of these materials were used against larvae of a number of mosquitoes. A 100 percent mortality rate was obtained against all larvae with the crude garlic extract at the concentration of 200 ppm or above, and 90 percent mortality if the concentration was 100 ppm. The steam distilled garlic oil fraction gave even better results: 100 percent mortality at 20 ppm for laboratory-bred larvae and 30 ppm for field-collected, highly insecticide-resistant larvae. They found that the oil fraction was 12 and one half times as effective as the crude garlic extract. Their research appeared in the *Journal of Economic Entomology* (63:1172, 1972).

Some of the various garlic preparations cited in Chapter 6 will be of use in reducing the itching, pain, and swelling accompanying insect bites and stings. These include fluid extract, fresh garlic juice, liniment, oil, ointment, and poultice. On the other hand, garlic capsules, pills, tablets, vinegar, and wine, when taken internally, help keep troublesome insects away. To actually kill them, one has to use the raw garlic as previously instructed.

LIP, MOUTH, AND THROAT PROBLEMS

Two physicians, D. M. Sergejev and I. D. Leonov, reported some years ago of treating 194 cases of lip and mouth disorders in a Soviet medical journal. They placed garlic paste on a gauze and applied it to the affected area, securing it in place with tape for eight to twelve hours. Complete healing was observed in over 90 percent of the cases in such disorders as leukoplakia (white spots), hyperkeratosis (a horny swelling), cold sores, fissures, and ulcers of the lips. See the next chapter under Poultice & Plaster for instructions on making a suitable paste.

Rufus Jordan of Lexington, Kentucky, told me some years ago what he did for cold sores. "I take a little smear of Vaseline, and put it on my lip. Then I take a piece of garlic clove, cut a slice of it, and lay the cut side right on the cold sore. The Vaseline helps to keep it from falling off. My sores disappear just like that," he finished with a snap of his fingers.

Matilda Sweet of Jonesboro, Arkansas, sent me the following remedy in 1972 for treating sore throats. "Make a garlic syrup by taking eight large cloves of garlic and smashing them into a paste. Add eight teaspoons of wine vinegar and stir. Leave overnight in the fridge for 24 hours to marinate. Warm two ounces of dark honey until it becomes quite liquid, then stir in six teaspoons of lime juice. When quite cool add this to the garlic paste and again stir well. Keep in a closed jar in the fridge until needed. For a sore throat, take two teaspoons and retain in the mouth until very liquid, then gently allow this to trickle down your throat, giving a little gargle now and then to bathe the back of the mouth and tonsils. Repeat thrice daily."

Two more remedies for treating cold sores and oral thrush came from Gladys Hogard in Northampton, England. For cold sores, she suggested mixing a level teaspoon of dried instant coffee with an equal amount of live-cultured yogurt into a paste. Then add two crushed cloves of garlic, about a tablespoon of honey, and enough cornmeal to thicken to a creamy base. Apply this to the affected area regularly. The mixture will eventually dry and fall off. When this happens, simply apply some more. This may not be the most attractive remedy if you're concerned about cosmetic appearances, but it does work, she claimed.

The second treatment is effective for soreness in the mouth from candida infection, ulcers on the gums, or soft tissues. Add two teaspoons of live-cultured yogurt to three crushed cloves of garlic and mix thoroughly. Take two teaspoons of this mixture, retaining it in your mouth and swishing it around the affected area with your tongue. It may sting a little at first but persevere. Keep this up for a few minutes and then spit out the mixture. Repeat three times daily. You will find some pain relief from this remedy and the condition will normally clear up within four to five days.

A cold garlic extract, decoction, electuary, essence, fluid extract, fomentation, juice, liqueur, ointment, and syrup would all be efficacious for lip, mouth, and throat problems.

LIVER DISEASE

Retired United States Air Force Major Edward Newman of San Francisco, sent me the following anecdote a few years back. "On October 17, 1966, I was hit with the first sign of real disease I have ever experienced. . . . A shockingly abrupt onset, with anorexia, nausea, fever, and malaise. Oh yes, you can throw in pruritus, urticaria, and intermittent diarrhea also. For the first time in my life I thought that I might die, and *that* was no joke, believe me! I remembered that a few weeks previously, I had been exposed to a 'recovered' Vietnam viral hepatitis patient, who had been let loose somewhat prematurely and was evidently another 'Typhoid Mary'. Since there was *no specific medical treatment* available, I followed the advice of my grandmother and chewed a large piece of garlic with a water chaser. Four pieces brought me back into the world of the living again, and I haven't been sick a day since making garlic part of my food supplement routine at the slightest hint of another liver infection."

The scientific literature certainly testifies to garlic's important value in treating liver disease. The *Japanese Journal of Nutrition* (26:74–78, 1968) reported that two sets of rats were fed a diet with rancid oil or rancid oil supplemented with a water extract of beef liver and Japanese aged garlic extract. Those with only the rancid oil had far heavier livers, and those with the liver-garlic extract had lighter livers with less fat in them.

Carbon tetrachloride is a poisonous chemical used in the dry cleaning industry, in fire extinguishers, as a solvent for oils and fats, as an insect exterminator, in spark plugs, and as a deworming agent in veterinary medicine. *The Merck Index* (Rahway, NJ: Merck & Co., Inc., 1976) 9th ed., warns: "Can be fatal ... primarily in liver damage ..." Because it is still so widely used, millions of people are exposed to trace amounts of it just about every day of their lives. Lengthy exposure can have very bad cumulative effects within the human liver.

Two published studies, based on the research of Shizutoshi Nakagawa and others, have shown that isolated compounds from Siberian ginseng root and Japanese aged garlic extract can effectively protect the liver from possible damage induced by carbon tetrachloride and other industrial chemicals.

"In general," Dr. Nakagawa wrote in the *Hiroshima Journal of Medical Sciences* (34:303–309, September, 1985), "sulphur-containing amino acids act as liver protective agents." In addition to garlic, onion, leek, and scallion, this group includes cabbage, kale, kohlrabi, cauliflower, mustard greens, watercress, horseradish, radish, and Brussels sprouts. All of these vegetables and herbs contain large amounts of sulphur protein, which helps protect the liver.

In *Phytotherapy Research* (1:1–4, 1988), which contained his second report, Dr. Nakagawa briefly explained how JAGE is made:

> Sliced raw garlic . . . is dipped into a 15 to 20 percent solution of ethanol over a long period of time (over 18 months) in a tank kept at room temperature. After the aging process, this garlic extract is then filtered and finally concentrated under low temperatures to eliminate the alcohol.

I should add here that in May and June of 1990, I went with some other scientists to Japan to see this aging process. The fields in northern Japan where this garlic comes from are meticulously prepared well in advance of its growth. The soil is enriched with sea vegetation and fish meal to insure a very potent garlic at harvest time. I cut off one of the green tops while out in the field and was casually munching on it when I suddenly felt an incredible need for water to quench the fiery feeling in my mouth. No regular green garlic top back home ever did this to me! Some of those in my group laughed good-naturedly at my unexpected "discovery" of the unbelievable strength of this particular garlic, which eventually goes through the aging process previously described.

In 1990, Padma P. Tadi, a doctoral student at Loma Linda University, presented an important paper at the Annual Meeting of The American Society For Microbiology held in Anaheim, California. Her study indicates that the use of JAGE in the diet may help prevent cancers caused by two chemicals, one of which is the leading cause of liver cancer, and the other, a chemical often found in cigarette smoke, charcoal-broiled meat, and polluted air.

Sulphur compounds of Japanese aged garlic extract were found to inhibit mutations caused by the potent liver carcinogen aflatoxin and the environmental pollutant benzo-[a]pyrene. Additionally, the JAGE compounds prevented the binding of aflatoxin to DNA and, at the same time, facilitated in the detoxification of the chemical.

Using an in vitro model with *Salmonella typhimurium* bacteria as the tester organism and rat liver enzymes for activation, the researchers demonstrated that two sulphur components from garlic (diallyl sulphide and ajoene) and JAGE could prevent the mutation induced by the two chemical carcinogens. These potential carcinogens require activation by liver enzymes before they are able to bind with DNA and exert their carcinogenic effects. The garlic compounds actually decreased the DNA damage caused by carcinogenic compounds and enhanced the enzyme activity involved in eliminating the liver carcinogen, aflatoxin.

Here's a great liver flush for protecting this organ against disease. Combine one pressed garlic clove, a tablespoon of pure virgin olive oil, and one tablespoon each of lemon and lime juice in a pint jar or thermos. Fill half full with hot water and shake thoroughly, then drink slowly on an empty stomach.

Garlic fluid extract, capsule, infusion, juice, oil, pill, syrup, tablet, tincture, vinegar, and wine all help to protect the liver to varying degrees.

PAIN

Dr. Ritchi Morris, a naturopathic physician and sports psychologist, has used Japanese aged garlic extract, Siberian ginseng, pangamic acid (of the B-complex group), and vitamin C for reducing the pain and swelling experienced by professional athletes when they injure muscle tissue, bone cartilage, and joints. Dr. Morris, who resides in Ardsley, New York, claims that garlic prevents fluid accumulation and lactic acid buildup in muscle tissue, which can cause pain and swelling.

In Oriental medicine, moxa, a fine downy herbal material, is frequently burned on the skin in a process called moxibustion to cauterize or to bring relief from muscular pains. Moxa specialists know various vital points on the skin that traditional science has shown to have special effects on the musculature, skeletal system, and internal organs.

The use of garlic will enhance the pain-relieving action of moxibustion. Place a slice of garlic about the size of a penny on a part of the body bothered with neuralgia or rheumatism. On top of this place a small amount of moxa, usually mugwort. Ignite it and allow it to smolder until the moxa burns itself out. Remove the garlic slice and rub a soothing calendula or comfrey salve on the skin if it has reddened from the heat. With plain moxa, three heat treatments are recommended; with garlic added, just one is sufficient.

Although less effective than moxibustion, the following will give some relief after being applied to the skin and covered with an electric heating pad: fluid garlic extract, friction (rubbing the area with several cut garlic cloves), juice, liniment, oil, ointment, and tincture.

RADIATION

A study conducted by Dr. Benjamin Lau of Loma Linda University School of Medicine and published in the

International Clinical Nutrition Review (9:27–31, January 1989) showed that when immune system white blood cells were first incubated in a dilute solution of Japanese aged garlic extract and then exposed to low levels of radiation, most of them survived intact. The cells not treated with Japanese aged garlic extract all died within 72 hours. In addition, many harmful cells that had been exposed to raw garlic juice perished in a matter of hours due to the effect of the fresh cloves.

Those working around instruments emitting low levels of radiation would certainly benefit from garlic capsules, tablets, or pills taken on a regular basis. This would include photocopy machines, medical x-ray equipment, microwave devices, computer terminals, and nuclear submarines.

RESPIRATORY DISEASES

The July 12, 1976, *Journal of the American Medical Association* reported that the reason residents of the Mediterranean are less prone to getting bronchitis than British residents, even though both areas have nearly equal humidity, is because the former consume huge amounts of garlic.

W. L. "Bill" Dauster, who moved to Humboldt, Kansas from Los Angeles at the age of 76 because of his emphysema, made himself grilled cheese sandwiches in which he put thin slices of raw garlic. This, he declared, helped him to breathe better than anything else. Garlic decoction, electuary, essence, infusion, liqueur, tincture, vinegar, and wine would all be helpful here.

STRESS

At the World Garlic Congress in 1990, Dr. Richard Kvetnansky of the Slovak Academy of Sciences in Bratislavia demonstrated how Japanese aged garlic extract dramatically lowered the stress-induced activation of the peripheral sympathetic system in stressed lab rodents.

An even more fascinating study on the effects of JAGE on mice exposed to various types of stress appeared in the Japanese journal *Oyo Yakuri Pharmacometrics* (28:991–1002, 1984). JAGE was tested for its effect on the physical conditions and behavior of mice exposed to four different stressors—four hour oscillation movement, rope climbing, 4° C. cold stimulus, and 40 percent alcohol administration. This effect was then compared with those of caffeine, glucose, and thiamine hydrochloride. It seems that JAGE accelerated recovery from fatigue induced by the exposure to four hour oscillation movement and prevented a decrease in physical strength induced by the exposure to four hour oscillation movement, chronic rope climbing, and prolonged cold stimulus. Additionally, JAGE was shown to counteract the inhibitory effect of alcohol on the acquisition of passive avoidance response and to accelerate the recovery from alcohol-induced incoordination in motor nerve activity in mice. JAGE accelerated the removal of blood alcohol in alcohol treated mice, too.

It would appear that raw garlic used in meal preparation, garlic decoction, infusion, capsule, tablet, pill, oil, or vinegar would all exhibit anti-stress activity to varying extents.

Finally, on a more humorous note, garlic can be terrific for relieving social and job pressures, if you don't mind being ostracized. Martin Donovan of Salem, Massachusetts wrote that he used garlic in the workplace for reducing stress. "I use at least three cloves of garlic a day. The result is that my boss will not come into my office to abuse me. When I go to a bank or retail store, my transactions are handled quickly and efficiently, even abruptly, and any questions or complaints I have are always promptly granted. Neighbors bid me hello from across the street or not at all. I am blissfully happy and healthy. The only people with whom I have any real contact are other garlic-eaters, and these are equally blissfully happy and healthy."

STEROID ABUSE

Steroid abuse among high school and college-age kids, professional athletes, and body-builders is pervasive throughout North America and Europe. This is a dangerous practice with serious life-threatening side effects. Garlic, believe it or not, can be a natural alternative to these harmful synthetic steroids.

According to *Chemical & Pharmaceutical Bulletin* (37:2741–43, 1989), garlic contains a number of naturally-occurring steroids. Some of these are growth hormones, and when garlic supplements were fed to domestic animals and chickens, it increased their overall weight. In a strange twist of irony, it was because of these few steroids in garlic that Canadian health officials temporarily seized batches of a garlic-based preparation used as a growth stimulant in pigs in the French Canadian province of Quebec. Farmers were understandably irate and the public even more furious. Eventually, the Ministry of Health had to relent and concede that garlic isn't a drug but a food spice, no matter how it's used.

According to the *Research Bulletin of the Punjab University* (11 [1–2]:37–47, June 1960), elephant garlic contains far more of these steroids than regular garlic does. Those seeking natural alternatives to steroids should consider eating more elephant garlic and taking extra supplements of Korean ginseng and sarsaparilla root, which are also known to contain trace amounts of steroids.

Garlic capsules, tablets, and pills may help give energy and prevent infection and muscle tissue injury, but it's doubtful they would supply any of the bulking steroids that raw elephant garlic or even green onions contain.

TOOTHACHE

A toothache usually signifies the presence of a cavity somewhere in the mouth. The scientific journal *Pharmazie* (38:747–48, 1983) mentioned a study in which volunteers rinsed their teeth after every meal using a mouthwash containing 10 percent garlic. They had significantly lower cavities than others who rinsed without the benefit of garlic. A garlic decoction or infusion is great for this.

As I described in Chapter 2, raw garlic makes an effective temporary treatment when an amalgam filling accidentally falls out and you're unable to get to your dentist right away.

A cotton ball soaked with some garlic cold extract or fluid extract may provide some relief, too, but I think the raw garlic works best in this situation.

WARTS

Dr. Henry Warren, a retired pathologist, gave me this handy remedy some time ago for getting rid of warts: Take a fresh clove of garlic and remove a thin slice across the clove with a razor blade or very sharp knife. Anoint the unaffected area immediately around the site of the wart with medicated petroleum jelly so that the garlic will not come into contact with it. Place the garlic on the wart and hold down with adhesive tape or a plaster. Apply a fresh slice daily. After a week to ten days the wart should come away completely.

A variation of this is to take a very ripe banana and peel it. Cut a square inch of the peel and turn it up with the yellow outside facing down. On top squeeze a little garlic juice or milky latex from a fresh dandelion stem. Apply this to the wart and fix in place with tape. Change the next morning with a fresh application. Repeat this procedure for seven to ten days, at which time the wart should have completely disappeared. (I am indebted to Dr. Mathew Midcap of Morganstown, West Virginia, for the banana peel suggestion.)

WORMS

A local Salt Lake City veterinarian told me that he sometimes mixes dehydrated garlic powder in the feed of cats he is treating for intestinal parasites. He claims that within three days or less, the worms are usually passed out of the system.

In Capetown and Johannesburg, South Africa, dogs frequently become infested with ticks during the summertime. Health-minded pet owners have found that giving small chopped pieces of garlic with their pets' chow will usually make the animal less attractive to ticks.

A letter in the *Medical Journal of Australia* (Jan. 23, 1982) from Dr. Rich of Adelaide recounted how he and all of his family were infected with ringworm by a stray kitten. His teenage daughter, the last to suffer, didn't think much of the antibiotic drug the others were using and decided to try garlic instead. Dr. Rich, being a scientist, persuaded her to treat one arm with garlic and the other with the modern drug. The lesions on her garlic-treated arm healed in only 10 days, while the other side took almost a month to clear up. A garlic fomentation, cold compress, liniment, ointment, or plaster would also be useful in treating ringworm or other fungal infections.

Omni magazine for September, 1979, mentioned several U.S. Government Health, Education and Welfare studies of urban and rural dwellers, showing they were hosts to intestinal parasites and that garlic was probably the best remedy for treatment.

William H. Khoe, M.D., of Ojai, California, routinely prescribes Japanese aged garlic extract capsules or tablets (three to five daily) for the removal of human parasites such as tapeworm, roundworm, and pinworm.

From the large amount of evidence presented, it is easy to see why garlic therapy is the right and proper choice for the management of many diseases and health problems.

CHAPTER SIX

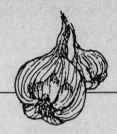

Garlic Preparations for Wellness and Recovery

A VARIETY OF FORMS

WHEN working with fresh garlic for medicinal purposes, it is important to keep in mind that the form in which this spice appears has a lot to do with its ultimate success or failure in treating a particular malady. You would certainly not pour garlic tea into the ear canal to treat an earache; a few drops of warm garlic oil would be much better. Nor would you smoke garlic in a pipe for a toothache; a natural packing of crushed garlic and peanut butter would work much better in reducing the pain and swelling until you get an appointment with your dentist.

In this chapter, 30 different preparations are carefully

described, as are the particular problems best suited for each application.

Some of these preparations are good only for immediate use (such as a warm garlic enema, used for treating a colicky or constipated infant), while others, which are alcohol-based, can last indefinitely under the right storage conditions in a cool, dry, dark place.

BATHS

The Romans were the first civilization to make full use of the mineral baths and hot springs available to them in the scattered parts of their vast empire. Here in the Western Hemisphere, the ancient Mayans developed an elaborate system of baths for similar purposes. Many centuries later, the Plains Indians and other North American tribes adapted the Mayan practice into the familiar sweatlodge ritual, complete with ceremonial accoutrements.

Full or partial garlic baths come in all sizes and shapes, from the bathtub to the eye cup. Basically, they are baths to which garlic teas have been added. The temperature often determines whether such a garlic bath will be calming or stimulating to the mind and body, whether it will open or close the pores of the skin, and whether it will relieve inflammation, pain, or itching.

When making a decoction (boiled tea) for adding to a full bath, anywhere from a few ounces to several pounds of garlic cloves may be tied or sewed into a linen or other cloth bag and then simmered in a quart to a gallon of water. For partial baths, the only difference is that smaller amounts are used, usually about a third as much as for a full bath. When taking the bath, you can put the bag into the water to extract more of the properties, and you can use it as an herbal "washcloth" to give yourself an invigorating rubdown.

Warm garlic baths should be around 95° F. (35° C.). They can be very calming and soothing to the nerves when combined with an equal amount of dried peppermint leaves. Warm garlic baths are especially helpful for bladder and urinary problems, colds, flus, and fevers. Both hot (100° F. or 43° C. to 113° F. or 45° C.) and cold (55° F. or 13° C. to 65° F. or 18° C.) garlic baths tend to shock the system in a positive way, causing increased heart action (in a cold garlic bath the heart slows down after the initial shock). The hot bath followed by bundling up in wool blankets will invariably induce profuse sweating and can be helpful for treating colds, flus, and fevers, not to mention eliminating body wastes retained because of improper kidney function. By adding other medicinal herbs to the full garlic bath, you can create a bath for just about any purpose you could imagine: to soften, moisturize, or scent the skin, to keep flying insects away in the summer, to remove excess oil, to relieve itching, to stimulate or relax, to tighten or tone the skin, to ease muscular aches, and many more. Don't be afraid to experiment with different herbs in conjunction with the garlic bath to find those that best suit your needs and purposes.

The half garlic bath is halfway between a full garlic bath and the garlic sitzbath. You can sit in water up to the navel with the legs and feet under water, but the upper portion of your body remains out of the water. A cold half garlic bath of no more than a minute and just once a day can be useful for migraines, insomnia, nervousness, overactive thyroid, intestinal gas, and constipation. The warm half garlic bath can be enjoyed somewhat longer, for ten minutes twice a day if necessary, once in the morning and again at night. It should be about 95° F. (35° C.) and can be used for lower back pain, low blood pressure, and menopausal difficulties. The warm half garlic bath usually includes a vigorous brushing of the skin with a natural bristle brush or luffa sponge and may be concluded with a brief spray of cold water on the back.

The garlic sitzbath involves sitting in a small amount of garlic water. To take a sitzbath, put enough warm or hot garlic bath water (actually garlic soup when you get right down to it) in the tub so that it reaches your navel. Prop your feet up on a hassock or chair beside the tub, then wrap yourself with large towels or blankets so you are completely covered from the neck down. If you are using a bathtub, put in about four inches of garlic water, keep your knees up, and splash the water onto your abdomen. Remain in the tub for half an hour, then rinse with a short cold bath or shower. Garlic sitzbaths are beneficial for the sexual reproductive organs and the urinary tract, the lower abdominal area, and the rectum. They are also of considerable value for remedying inflammations, pelvic congestion, cramps, hemorrhoids, menstrual problems, and kidney and intestinal pains.

For a garlic footbath, simply place your feet and calves into a deep pot or tub filled with plain garlic water. For coldness in the lower extremities, a hot garlic footbath for half an hour makes a good treatment. It has also been recommended by skilled herbalists for bladder, kidney, throat, and ear inflammations.

Sometimes the exact opposite may work wonders. Consider the case of the man who made headlines some time ago in Altoona, Pennsylvania. He claimed he cured all of his colds and flus simply by immersing his two big toes in ice cold garlic water for an average of three minutes daily. He made a strong, clear garlic soup, then placed it in the freezer until it was sufficiently chilled without being frozen. Some have claimed that cold (but not frigid) garlic footbaths are good for tired feet, constipation, headache, and nosebleed. Some of my students and I have tried this for the above conditions and found it to have worked for all of them except constipation.

By alternating between hot and cold garlic footbaths, circulation in the lower extremities is definitely improved, varicose veins are helped, and even weak menstrual flow is increased. Insomnia, migraine, hypertension, and persistently cold feet are assisted as well. First soak the feet in the hot garlic bath for two minutes, then place them in the cold garlic bath for no more than 30 seconds, then start over again. Alternate between the two baths for 20 minutes, always making sure you end with the cold.

Maurice Mességué, one of Europe's greatest folk healers and herbalists, often treated kings, queens, popes, dictators, artists, musicians, and other dignitaries with nothing more than foot and hand baths used together. His lengthy practice enabled him to confirm the virtues of such garlic baths for successfully treating allergies, asthma, acne (associated with stomach and intestinal problems), and hypertension.

Mességué gave instructions for preparing the full, half, foot, and hand garlic baths in his popular French bestseller, *Health Secrets of Plants and Herbs* (N.Y.: William Morrow & Co., Inc., 1979). He attributed the recipe for these baths to his grandmother Sophie, who passed it on to his father. Take 30 cloves of garlic and slightly bruise them. Pour over them about three gallons of boiling water. Cover with a lid and let stand in a big plastic or metal bucket for half a day. Reheat this entire amount in several large pots until sufficiently hot again, then strain through a colander or large wire sieve into the bathtub and fill the tub with more hot tap water to the desired depth. For half baths, simply cut the above amounts of garlic and water by 50 percent; for sitzbaths, reduce them to 30 percent and for hand and foot baths, cut to just 15 percent. Mességué mentioned that it is not necessary to dilute sitz, hand, or foot baths with extra tap water.

There is also the vapor bath, which is particularly suited for inhalation. The simplest form of the vapor bath, which is also called aromatherapy now, is to hang a sachet filled with cloves of garlic about the neck during episodes of colds, influenza, tuberculosis, or other respiratory diseases until the problem is resolved. For an inhalant garlic vapor bath, you need a chair, a pot containing a steaming garlic tea, something to set the pot on, and enough blankets to enclose you and the entire works completely.

To make the necessary garlic tea, first bruise several cloves of garlic and place them in a small saucepan with just enough water to cover. Simmer gently with the lid on over low heat for about 20 minutes. Leave covered and allow to cool down only enough so that the resulting steam won't damage the mucus linings of the nose and sinus cavities. Add one teaspoon lemon or lime juice to this solution and stir. It is important to keep the pot covered at all times so that valuable steam doesn't escape and cool down too quickly.

Next, arrange the chair and the pot so that you can hold your head over the pot to inhale the garlic vapors. Have someone else drape blankets all around so that you and the pot are entirely enclosed. An easier version is to have the pot resting on a low table or counter top with your head directly above it by several inches and a blanket or large towel draped over everything.

With your head above the pot by several inches, breathe the garlic vapor for 15 minutes. This can sometimes be accompanied by a cold garlic sitz or half bath lasting just a few minutes, followed by a few hours in bed, warmly wrapped in blankets like a mummy. This garlic vapor bath is ideal for colds, flus, sinus and respiratory problems, and inner ear inflammations.

The sauna really provides the most ideal garlic vapor bath, but not everyone is so fortunate as to have one. Since necessity is the mother of invention, one can improvise by building his or her own. A cane chair (one with holes in the seat) is required, along with two pots of steaming garlic tea, a wooden grate, and enough blankets to enclose everything, including you, from the neck or waist down. Place one pot beneath the chair and the other directly in front of it so that you can comfortably rest your feet on the wooden grate when it is placed on top of this second pot. Sit on the chair, put your feet on the grate, and have someone else enclose you and the pots completely. You need to be enclosed just from the waist down, but it may be easier to make a good seal at the neck as well. This particular garlic vapor bath lasts about half an hour, and should be followed by a cold garlic half bath of no more than a minute. The final part of the treatment is bed, as with the inhalant vapor bath. The vapor bath is good for kidney and intestinal pains and for prostate problems. If you have cystitis or prostatitis, omit the cold garlic half bath.

To make a sufficiently hot garlic tea for this homemade sauna treatment, follow the preceding instructions but double the ingredients and the time for cooking.

Be advised that garlic should *never* come into direct contact with the eyes because of its highly irritating sulphur fumes. If an allergic skin reaction occurs with any of these baths, discontinue at once and consult a dermatologist or allergist.

For those not ambitious enough to peel the raw cloves necessary for making a full or half bath, one half to one cup of garlic powder or more can be used in a half tub of hot water. Buy your garlic powder in bulk at any health food or herb store for this purpose.

BOLUS

The chief difference between a garlic bolus and a suppository is that the former is for insertion into the vagina for treating vaginitis and similar infections and the latter is for insertion into the anus to help with hemorrhoids.

Powdered garlic is made into a thick clay-like consistency using melted cocoa butter, water, or honey and then placed in the refrigerator just long enough to harden, after which it is removed and allowed to warm to room temperature before use. It is rolled into strips about three-quarters of an inch thick and cut into segments about an inch in length. When water is used in place of cocoa butter, place the formed boluses on a cookie sheet in the oven at a low temperature of 120° F. (49° C.). When they are dry and hard you can store them in an airtight jar.

The best time to insert the bolus is at night just before retiring. The cocoa butter will melt due to the body heat, releasing the garlic into the system. Garlic seems to be most effective at night. When inserting a water-based bolus into the vagina, use a little lotion or petroleum jelly as a lubricant for easy insertion. When honey is used as the moistening agent, just mix a small amount of it with the garlic powder to make a very stiff clay-like consistency. Form it and then stiffen by storing in the refrigerator. Although a honey bolus can work very well, it will not be as firm as the other two types, though it is usually firm enough for vaginal use.

CAPSULE

See GELATIN CAPSULE.

COLD COMPRESS

Soak a cotton cloth or terry hand towel in cool garlic tea, wring out the excess liquid, and apply to any part of the body that is inflamed due to sunburn, windburn, or sunstroke. Try to keep the cold garlic compress away from the eyes, if applying it to the forehead. Leave on until it is warmed by body heat, which takes about 20 minutes. Repeat the application with a fresh cool garlic compress and continue until relief is obtained. This also works well with sciatica, neuralgia, and toothache when alternated, hot and cold. It can also be of great help in reducing the pain and swelling of a sprained or twisted ankle, pulled muscle ligament, injured kneecap, sore wrist or elbow, and so forth.

COLD EXTRACT

A garlic preparation made with ordinary cold water will help to preserve the herb's volatile and essential oils, water-soluble vitamins, and sulphur salts. Cover several bruised garlic cloves with cold water, being sure to use an enamelled pan, wooden bowl, or plastic container instead of a metallic pot. Let the mixture stand a good 16 hours in a cool, dark area, then strain, and the drink is ready. Alternatively, combine six or eight garlic cloves with two cups cold water in a blender. Blend at high speed for a few seconds, let mixture stand overnight, strain, and use.

DECOCTIONS

A decoction is a simmered tea. When you wish to extract primarily the sulphur and other valuable mineral salts from garlic (rather than the vitamins and volatile ingredients), decoction is the best way to go. For every quarter teaspoon of coarsely chopped garlic clove, use about one and a quarter cups of water in an enamelled pot. Bring the water to a rolling boil first, then add the garlic. Reduce the heat and simmer uncovered for no more than five minutes. Then remove from the heat, cover with a lid, and steep for 45 minutes. Strain and drink in half cup amounts.

Both garlic decoctions and infusions are handy for a variety of respiratory ailments and bacterial and viral infections. Because they can be so potent, however, they should be taken in small amounts spread out over many hours each day. (See also INFUSION.)

DOUCHE

A garlic douche is the best treatment for vaginal infections or cleansing the body. However, garlic douches shouldn't be overused as they can upset the delicate balance of natural flora within the vagina itself. A garlic douche is made by preparing a strong decoction. After the decoction has steeped for awhile, add a tablespoon of apple cider vinegar or garlic vinegar to help promote acid balance within the vagina. The douche is best applied in an empty bathtub or on the toilet, but never have the douche bag more than two feet above the hips. The garlic douche is slowly and gently inserted while still warm (at body temperature) and retained for up to half an hour, if possible. If the liquid is forced in under too much pressure, it may push the infection upward towards the uterus. Don't douche if you are pregnant.

ELECTUARY

An electuary is an old-fashioned way of giving garlic to sick children who may require a strong but natural antibiotic of some kind. A small amount of finely minced garlic is mixed with either dark honey, blackstrap molasses, pure maple syrup, organic peanut butter, or some other tasty medium until a soft pasty mass is formed. The sick child is then given this to eat in small amounts. The sweet flavor will encourage a willingness to consume the garlic without much fuss.

ENEMA

A lukewarm garlic enema can be administered in cases of stomach flu, intestinal parasites, or constipation. A garlic infusion is usually prepared for this, but in some cases something stronger, such as a garlic decoction, may be necessary.

A garlic enema is taken in while first lying on the right side, then on hands and knees, and finally lying on the left side. This will help the solution to fill the lower intestines better. The garlic fluid should be retained for as long as possible and the procedure repeated every few hours or until two quarts of garlic decoction have been taken in and retained for several minutes at a time. The bathroom is the best place for doing this. Lay some newspaper down on the floor and fill a hot water bottle two-thirds full of warm garlic decoction. Make sure a hose with a syringe attachment is put on tight. Hang the apparatus up on a clothes hook or run the hole at the top through 3 or 4 wire hangers suspended from the shower curtain rod. Apply some olive oil or petroleum jelly to the end of the syringe and insert into the rectum while in a flat position on the floor. Don't take in more than what your body is capable of retaining.

ESSENCE

Dissolve one tablespoon of homemade garlic oil in a pint of vodka or brandy. This is a good way to preserve garlic's more volatile compounds, some of which aren't soluble in water. It's also handy for rubbing across the forehead for migraines or on the sides of the face and throat for neuralgia and sore throat. Be careful to keep it out of your eyes. An essence is for external application.

FLUID EXTRACT

A fluid extract should never be confused with a tincture. A commercial fluid extract is made by techniques that utilize multiple solvent extraction and can take up to a month or more to complete. This results in a very concentrated product that is often up to ten times as potent as a tincture and, therefore, only taken in small quantities, such as six to eight drops at a time. The recommended amount of tincture is often double or triple these figures. A fluid extract is so concentrated that it should always be diluted with water or juice before taking.

Special equipment and training are needed to make a commercial fluid extract of garlic. The process requires several gallons of an appropriate solvent such as vodka, several hundred cloves of raw garlic, and an elevated container large enough to accommodate these materials. The cloves have to be macerated and the entire material cold-percolated with as little heat as possible in order to retain most of the active principles. A very slow drip method through connecting hoses or pipes into a secondary container of smaller size is employed to get the final fluid extract, after which the menstruum or original extraction materials are discarded.

Sometimes a fluid extract of garlic that has reached this stage may be subjected to further purification processes to eliminate unnecessary fats or oily resins with additional solvents. The term "purified garlic extract" is used to identify this secondary extraction.

The benefits of a commercially prepared fluid extract of garlic derive from its strength. It is strong enough to combat even the most stubborn of the infectious viruses, that have become resistant to synthetic antibiotics. German and French research chemists have shown that otherwise hardy viruses can be easily vanquished by potent commercial fluid extracts of garlic. Health food stores usually carry the milder and more common garlic tinctures, which are sometimes mislabelled "fluid extracts." Most European herb shops and botanical pharmacies carry various brands of the more powerful fluid extract of garlic. Those travelling abroad would do well to visit stores in the United Kingdom, France, Austria, Belgium, Germany, and the Netherlands to purchase liquid garlic extracts. Some naturopathic doctors in the U.S. and Canada may also carry these potent garlic extracts in their arsenal of materia medica.

An old work from 1908, *A Practical Treatise on Materia Medica and Therapeutics* (Philadelphia: F. A. Davis Co., 1908) by John V. Shoemaker, M.D., gave as the standard rule of strength for such fluid extracts this formula: "1,000 cubic centimetres of the fluid extract represents the active principle of 1,000 grams of the crude drug."

FOMENTATION

A garlic fomentation is an external wet application to treat skin infections, open sores, wounds, swellings, and respiratory ailments in the chest. It is similar in some ways to a garlic poultice but is usually weaker and therefore less dramatic in its actions. Some practicing herbalists equate a compress with a fomentation.

To make a fomentation, make a garlic tea in advance. Take a very moisture-absorbent cotton cloth or terry towel, dip it into the hot garlic tea, wring out the excess liquid, and apply immediately to the area of the body desired. The wet material should be covered by a dry flannel cloth and a heating pad or hot water bottle. This keeps the heat in for a longer period of time. A plastic covering is used to protect bedding if it is to be applied overnight.

FRICTION

Maurice Mességué, a famous French herbalist and popular European health writer, recommended that his older male patients who suffered from impotence rub some garlic on the tailbone near the base of the spine. Several cloves of garlic are peeled and slightly flattened with a heavy object; they are then firmly grasped between the fingers and rubbed in a circular motion in this area for about 10 minutes every day. Mességué claimed a 35 to 45 percent success rate for impotence with this method.

GELATIN CAPSULE

Most manufactured single-herb or formula products sold in the health food industry today are in gelatin capsules. They are inexpensive to produce, convenient for consumers to take, and more easily digested than tablets. Capsules should be stored at all times in a cool, dry place and kept away from heat and humidity. Their average shelf life is about three years.

Both garlic oil and garlic powder can be put into capsules, then placed in heavy plastic or dark glass bottles which are light and moisture resistant. Manufacturers apply tamper-proof seals before airtight lids are screwed on.

Though intended for internal consumption, such capsules are versatile and can also be opened and used for external purposes. Between 6 to 10 capsules may be required to equal a level teaspoon of garlic oil or powder.

Garlic capsules should be taken at night just before retiring in order to obtain maximum benefits. To eliminate the noticeable garlic odor on the breath, take the capsules with a meal, several parsley tablets, fresh parsley and peppermint, or a mixed green drink (dark leafy greens and carrot juice). With the odorless forms of garlic now available, odor is no longer a problem, although some consumers may have to try more than one brand to find a product that is truly odorless for them. Individual reactions vary.

Garlic capsules offer nearly the same antibiotic advantages that synthetic pharmaceuticals do for many kinds of infections. For disease prevention, an average of two capsules daily is recommended. For treating serious illnesses like hepatitis or cancer, triple this amount twice daily may be necessary.

Garlic capsules are also good for bringing down elevated serum cholesterol and triglyceride levels. Usually about four a day is adequate. In cases of early arteriosclerosis, though, double this amount may be advisable.

Because garlic is strongly hypoglycemic, it is of proven benefit to those suffering from insulin-dependent diabetes. As few as six and as many as 10 capsules per day may be taken with good results. However, those with the opposite problem, low blood sugar or hypoglycemia, should experiment first with just one or two capsules to make sure there are no unpleasant reactions to the garlic, such as fatigue, mood swings, nervousness, depression, anxiety, forgetfulness, or insomnia. In this case, the garlic should be discontinued and other herbs tried instead.

In 1990 I asked Benjamin Lau, M.D., Ph.D., a professor of microbiology and internal medicine at Loma Linda Medical School, if he had ever found problems with garlic in his hypoglycemic patients. His response was that there were occasional problems with raw garlic, but never when they took aged garlic extract.

INFUSION

When you want a milder garlic broth or tea, an infusion is the way to go. Unlike a decoction, which requires boiling, an infusion is simply steeped. Generally, between one and three macerated cloves are steeped in a pint of boiling water in a tightly covered enamel, porcelain, or glass pot away from the stove. Steeping in this manner usually occupies no more than 20 minutes, but it can take longer if desired.

A novel variation calls for putting several peeled and macerated cloves of raw garlic into a glass pint jar, filling it two-thirds full with spring or distilled water, screwing the lid on tightly, and setting it in the sun for half a day. This makes a wonderful infusion.

Making an infusion rather than a decoction preserves more heat-sensitive nutrients such as vitamin C. Also, an infusion is better for very young children and the recuperating elderly. An infusion is preferred to a decoction when administering an enema to an infant or child. (See also DECOCTION.)

JUICE

Maurice Mességué sometimes used full-strength garlic juice for very stubborn infections or fungal growths which had become drug resistant. He pressed several garlic cloves into a pulp and strained the juice through a fine cloth. Then he added the same amount of 90-proof alcohol and 10 times the amount of distilled water. This is a strong antiseptic and keeps indefinitely.

LINIMENT

A garlic liniment that includes some eucalyptus oil quickly penetrates the pores of the skin and is ideal for treating strained muscles and ligaments. It can also be used for the relief of rheumatoid arthritis, psoriasis, lupus erythematosus, and similar inflammations. This combination brings a relaxing warmth to tense muscles and expands the blood vessels to increase the flow of circulation.

Peel and slightly bruise four cloves of fresh garlic. Put them into a quart jar. Add two and a half cups of apple cider vinegar and a half cup of gin. Seal with a lid and set aside in a cool, dry place to extract. Shake the contents of the jar three times daily, morning, noon, and night. This process will take about two weeks to complete. Strain and discard the cloves, then add 15 to 20 drops of eucalyptus oil. Shake well and reseal until needed.

The use of the vinegar and alcohol causes the liniment to feel cool and evaporate quickly, leaving no messy residue behind. The aromatic eucalyptus oil guarantees fast penetration and rapid relief.

LIQUEUR

Maurice Mességué, the renowned French folk healer, made the following liqueur from garlic and gave it to some of his older patients as an occasional tonic for increasing their vitality. In a quart fruit jar put five crushed cloves of fresh garlic and three cups red burgundy wine. Seal with a lid and set on the window sill so it is exposed to plenty of sunlight for fourteen days. Shake every so often. Strain through fine cheesecloth and rebottle in a dark glass bottle with a tight-fitting lid. Take two drops the first day, four the second, six the third and so on until you reach 24; then reverse the procedure until you arrive back at two again.

OIL

Homemade garlic oil is one of the finest household remedies to have around. It is especially valuable for infants and young children for the treatment of earaches, inner ear infections, teething, thrush (oral candida), diaper rash, athlete's foot, genital itch, bed sores, and minor burns. Garlic oil will keep its intended potency for up to three months if properly stored in a dark glass bottle with a tight-fitting lid inside the refrigerator. To avoid rancidity, be sure to refrigerate and add a few drops of eucalyptus oil or glycerine as a preservative. For convenience, use a dropper bottle. One teaspoon of garlic oil is equivalent to one clove garlic.

Finely mince enough fresh garlic cloves to equal three quarters of a cup of garlic. Put into a large wooden or plastic mixing bowl and add three quarters of a cup of pure virgin olive oil. Add the oil slowly a quarter cup at a time while stirring. Put in a covered glass jar and set on the window still where it can get lots of sunshine. Let it stand for one and a half weeks. Shake the jar gently two or three times a day. On the eleventh day, strain the contents through several layers of cheesecloth and store the oil in the refrigerator. To avoid rancidity, be sure to refrigerate and add a few drops of eucalyptus oil or glycerine as a preservative.

To warm a little of the oil for dropping into the ear to relieve an earache or treat an inner ear infection in a young child, put about six to eight drops on a clean teaspoon. Hold a candle under it or hold the spoon over a gas burner for no more than a minute, until the oil becomes lukewarm and pleasant when dropped on the back of the hand. Place the oil in an empty dropper. With the child's head tilted sideways, place the dropper close to the opening of the ear and gently squeeze three to four drops into the ear. More can be added later on, but do not put too much (more than eight drops) into the child's ear at any one time.

OINTMENT

An old-fashioned garlic ointment made in Hong Kong some years ago by an aging Chinese herbalist is useful for any external skin infections or oral problems such as cold sores. One whole garlic bulb and its cloves are peeled and coarsely chopped, then placed in one pint of hot water. It is boiled, uncovered on low heat long enough to permit half of the water to evaporate. The remaining liquid is then strained into a hot cup of olive oil, vegetable shortening, or petroleum jelly. Some beeswax is slowly added afterwards until a firm consistency is obtained. A little gum benzoin or tincture of benzoin added just before the mixture becomes stiff helps preserve the ointment longer.

PACKING

A unique garlic packing devised by herbalist Lalitha Thomas has proven very helpful in treating open sores, major wounds, bad cuts, skin fissures, insect bites and stings, animal bites and scratches, and similar injuries.

Her remedy calls for equal parts of powdered slippery elm, garlic, and myrrh, mixed together dry in a large bowl. Then enough raw, uncooked honey, aloe vera gel, glycerin, or blackstrap molasses is added to make a smooth, even paste. This material is packed into or upon any part of the skin in need of soothing and healing. It works well for sunburn, other minor burns, and general inflammation.

PILL

Garlic pills are used in much the same way as garlic capsules, but they have the added advantage of not being affected by heat so they last longer. Peel five cloves of garlic

and finely mince them. Add a small amount of powdered
slippery elm bark and powdered marshmallow root (equal
parts), not to exceed 10 percent of the mixture. Slowly add
distilled or spring water and mix it with the garlic and powdered herbs until a doughy consistency has been achieved,
or use a little gum arabic dissolved in boiling water as an
adhesive. Roll the dough into little balls about the size of a
pea. The pills may be taken immediately, but to preserve
them for later use, dry them in the warm air or in an oven
on a cookie sheet at low heat for 30 minutes or longer. These
pea-sized pills contain about one-quarter the dose of a gelatin capsule, so you would need to take approximately four
of them to equal a capsule. Such pills are taken for all of
the same uses listed under gelatin capsules.

POULTICE AND PLASTER

A garlic poultice is a warm, moist mass of either
powdered or well-macerated cloves that is applied directly
to the skin for treating blood poisoning, venomous bites,
disease eruptions (measles, mumps, chickenpox), insect
stings, rose bush or cat scratches, slivers, genital herpes, ve-
nereal disease, Kaposi sarcoma (common with AIDS victims), and so forth.

It is a good idea to add a little finely grated fresh ginger
root or a pinch of powdered cayenne pepper to the garlic
to promote better circulation. It is also necessary to add a
small amount of a mucilaginous herb such as comfrey root,
marshmallow root, or slippery elm powder for adhesion.

The garlic and powdered herbs can be moistened with
hot black or green tea or a tincture of witch hazel, available
from any pharmacy. Spread this moistened paste or pulp on
a wet, hot wash cloth, apply with the plant material against
the skin, and then cover with another dry cloth in order to

keep the moisture and heat inside as long as possible. The first cloth can be moistened from time to time with additional teaspoons of hot water before being covered up again.

A simpler version of this calls for the raw cloves of garlic to be peeled and macerated, then applied directly to the skin with nothing over them. Because raw garlic may cause blistering in some cases, test a small area first.

A plaster is similar to a poultice, but the pounded garlic mass is either placed between two thin pieces of linen or combined in a thick base with powdered herbs before being applied to the skin.

An old-fashioned garlic-mustard plaster, though somewhat irritating to the skin, is ideal for aches, sprains, pulled ligaments, spasms, lower back pain, sciatica, and coldness in the extremities. It is made by combining equal parts of powdered yellow mustard and garlic powder with just enough tincture of witch hazel to make a thick paste. The paste is spread on a cotton cloth. Another thin cloth is placed on the skin and the mustard cloth put over that. The plaster should remain on until the skin begins to redden and a burning sensation is felt. The plaster is removed and the residue is washed away with cold water.

This plaster shouldn't be used on tender, sensitive areas of the body, such as around the eyes or the groin area. If the mustard powder seems too strong, it can be cut with a little rye or whole wheat flour. After removing this plaster, the skin should be powdered with rice flour, whole wheat flour, or powdered slippery elm bark, then wrapped with dry cotton.

Another excellent way to cool the skin following the application of a garlic-mustard plaster is to use tofu. Put some tofu in a cheesecloth bag or fine-mesh wire strainer and squeeze all of the excess water out of it. Then mash the tofu together with 20 percent pastry flour and 5 percent grated fresh ginger root. This is applied directly to the skin for cooling off the area.

POWDER

There are advantages and disadvantages to using commercially prepared garlic powder for remedial means. On the plus side, a powder is much easier to work with than are macerated, wet, pulpy cloves. The powder can be mixed with any type of liquid and formed into paste, poultice, plaster, pills, and tablets. The down side is that if high heat was used to create the powder, valuable vitamins, minerals, enzymes, and fats may have been lost, thereby reducing some of the garlic's healing powers.

To make your own garlic powder, peel and coarsely chop fresh cloves of garlic, spread them on a cookie sheet, and place in an oven at a low heat for several hours, until thoroughly dried. To preserve as many nutrients as possible, you can avoid heat altogether and dry garlic at room temperature in dry weather by spreading chopped garlic on cheesecloth spread over wire racks near a fan or strong breeze. Grind the dried garlic in a coffee grinder or spice mill. The resulting garlic powder should be kept in an airtight glass or plastic container and stored in a dry, cool place.

SALVE

A salve is synonymous with ointment.

SMOKING

Of all the ways in which garlic can be used, this is perhaps the strangest. But when combined with other herbs and smoked, garlic is efficacious in three specific areas: relieving coughs, clearing up bronchial congestion, and relieving the addiction to tobacco.

The best way to smoke garlic with other herbs is in a pipe or in self-rolled cigarette paper. For bronchial congestion, smoking garlic in combination with coltsfoot and mullein leaves will bring great relief. This is especially true for asthma sufferers. For the relief of a hacking cough, smoking garlic with peppermint leaves and rosemary herb will yield satisfying results.

To aid in quitting the tobacco habit, lobelia (also known as Indian tobacco) is smoked with garlic. It contains lobeline, which is similar to nicotine but doesn't have the same effects. Lobeline and some of the aromatic sulphur components in garlic will reduce the sensation of need for nicotine, but they don't themselves lead to addictive smoking.

Mugwort and catnip have been smoked with garlic in India, China, and Great Britain because of their calming effects in treating insomnia and restlessness. They also tend to reduce some of the stress and nervousness which prompts people to smoke in the first place.

To make garlic suitable for smoking, here are some simple directions. First, peel and coarsely chop the cloves in two bulbs of raw, whole garlic. Spread these evenly on a cookie sheet and set in the oven on low heat for several hours until they are thoroughly dried. Allow them to stand on a counter or stove top overnight until all moisture is gone.

Spread half of them on a clean white cloth or dish towel and cover with the remaining portion. With a rolling pin, go back and forth several times over these dried garlic pieces to reduce them in size a little more. Be careful not to roll too many times, because you don't want powder but rather particles about the size of BB shot.

At this stage, combine the garlic with some of the dried herbs previously mentioned. The entire mixture is then ready for smoking. Some of it can be tapped into a pipe (I'm told that corncob pipes seem to work best for this), or a sheet of tobacco paper can be used.

Smoking herbs in this manner is strictly for medicinal purposes and not intended for pleasure or smoking satisfaction. Smoking is a bad habit and should be avoided whenever possible. But the use of garlic in conjunction with other herbs in this manner is medically relevant when other treatments may have failed.

SUPPOSITORY

A garlic suppository is for insertion into the anus, for treating hemorrhoids or anal infections. AIDS victims often suffer from severe anal infections and garlic suppositories will be of great value to them. To make a garlic suppository, consult the section under BOLUS in this chapter and follow the instructions given there, using either cocoa butter or water. Shape the suppository for easy insertion into the anus.

SYRUP

Garlic syrup is a great way to administer garlic to young children and the elderly in cases of coughing, laryngitis, sore throat, or tonsillitis. There are two basic garlic syrups from which to choose.

Syrup #1 calls for half a cup of peeled, finely minced raw cloves of garlic placed into a small stainless steel, glass, or enamelled cooking pot. Add enough raw dark honey or blackstrap molasses to cover the garlic and very slowly simmer on low heat until the garlic seems to have disappeared into the syrup, about 20 minutes. Cover the pot to lessen the evaporation of essential nutrients, but stir frequently with a wooden spoon to avoid burning. While simmering, the syrup can be diluted with distilled or spring water, if you wish. Strain (if you don't like the garlic bits left in) and store in the refrigerator. This syrup can be used as frequently as you want. It is commonly taken as needed or every hour in teaspoon doses for small children and tablespoon doses for teenagers and adults.

Prepare syrup #2 the same as you would #1. Depending upon your need, add any or all of the following to the garlic and honey or molasses:

—1 teaspoon cloves (whole or powdered) for pain relief.
—1½ tablespoons slippery elm bark or marshmallow root (powdered) for additional decongesting and healing of injured throat and lung tissues.
—1½ tablespoons grated fresh ginger root or 1 teaspoon dried ginger root powder for increasing overall circulation, warmth, and effectiveness of the syrup.

Both of these syrups were originally devised by my friend Lalitha Thomas of Prescott, Arizona, with onion as the chief ingredient. I adapted them to garlic and have used the syrups successfully in a number of cases.

TABLET

Some herbal manufacturers still make garlic tablets. Tablets are handy because they do not deteriorate in heat as gelatin capsules do, so in hot and humid parts of the world, such as the jungles of Central America or Indonesia, where I've done my share of trekking, they are preferable to capsules.

Unfortunately, compression and heat are required to mold and bake these tablets, which destroys some of the garlic's valuable enzymes and vitamins. You need to take about three garlic tablets for every garlic capsule to get the same strength.

TEA

(See DECOCTION and INFUSION)

TINCTURE

A garlic tincture is similar to a fluid extract of garlic, only not as potent. It is used for exactly the same conditions that are treated by a fluid extract of garlic. (See FLUID EXTRACT.)

To make a good garlic tincture, peel and coarsely chop four to five cloves of raw garlic. Place them in one pint of vermouth, vodka, gin, brandy, or rum. Shake twice daily, morning and evening, to agitate the contents and expedite the extraction process. Do this for a maximum of 21 days, then filter the fluid through a strain or cheesecloth.

Michael Tierra, a practicing herbalist in Santa Cruz, California, recommends that all herbal tinctures be made "on the new moon and strained off on the full moon so that the drawing power of the waxing moon will help extract the herbal properties."

Had my own Hungarian grandmother, Barbara Liebhardt Heinerman, not done this herself years ago, I would have suspected this piece of advice. But having experimented with making garlic tincture by different lunar phases, I can attest to the stronger properties of the new moon garlic tincture. I attribute this, in part, to the earth's electromagnetic forces as well as the moon's gravitational pull.

Average intake for a garlic tincture should be between

10 to 15 drops once or twice daily, as needed. Because it's weaker than a fluid extract of garlic, this tincture doesn't need to be diluted in water or juice but can be taken straight underneath the tongue.

VINEGAR

Maurice Mességué, the great French folk healer, often used garlic vinegar for disinfecting bed sores, diabetic leg ulcers, wounds, skin conditions such as scabies and ringworm, and the successful removal of corns, warts (general, genital, and anal), and callouses.

To make garlic vinegar, he would peel and macerate three cloves of grated garlic in three and a half cups of wine vinegar (apple cider vinegar may be substituted) for two weeks. To treat the sores, ulcers, and wounds, he applied a cold compress of this garlic vinegar and left it on the affected part until it became warm from body heat, then replaced it with another fresh cold one. For scabies and ringworm, he would wash the skin with the vinegar, rubbing it with a coarse cloth to help it soak in faster. He would usually add two drops of camphorated oil to the garlic vinegar for this purpose, in order to open the pores of the skin.

The best way to use this remedy for getting rid of corns, warts, and callouses is to soak a small cotton ball with garlic vinegar, gently squeeze out the excess, then tape it directly to the growth, leave it on overnight, and change it again the next morning.

WINE

There are two types of garlic wine, both of which are useful in cases of fever, intestinal parasites, and general physical weakness. The first is of French origin and was used extensively by Mességué in his practice. He peeled and slightly bruised a whole bulb of garlic and put it into a stone crock or glass jar with 10 pinches of fresh and finely cut wormwood leaves. To this he added three and a half cups of hot red or white wine and let it set for five days. The dose was two wine glassfuls (a total of four fluid ounces) a day.

A favorite household remedy in some American and Canadian Chinatowns and also in Hong Kong is a garlic wine kept handy for the cold and flu season. The wine is prepared by soaking three peeled garlic bulbs in one cup of uncooked rice wine for at least one month. Whoever catches a cold or flu takes a tablespoon of this mixture every two hours and again just before retiring. To minimize the undesirable flavor, some Chinese dissolve a little white sugar in boiling water and add this to the garlic wine. But, since sugar isn't good for you, particularly when you are sick, this practice is discouraged.

CHAPTER SEVEN

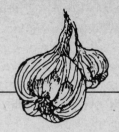

World Garlic Festivals

GARLIC festivals can be fun and informative for the garlic aficionado. Following are some of my favorites.

GARLIC FESTIVAL, GILROY, CALIFORNIA

Gilroy, California, is a place that American humorist Will Rogers once described as "the only town where you can marinate a steak by hanging it out on the clothesline." In 1979 a group of local residents staged the first weekend celebration of the "scented pearl" to promote a positive image of the community. Yearly attendance has grown from a modest 20,000 to over 150,000. This festival has made headlines the world over.

The heart of this huge and well-run festival is Gourmet Alley, where local chefs perform culinary magic over the firepits in full view of the spectators. While Gourmet Alley's volunteer chefs create delicious delights, other clubs and civic groups present an impressive array of international garlic dishes that make this the granddaddy of all garlic extravaganzas.

The heart and soul of this festival are booths with delicious garlic bread, garlic soup, calamari, scampi, garlic buttered corn, even garlic beer and garlic ice cream! Garlic gimmicks being sold may include garlic hats, t-shirts, wine glasses, jewelry and pet garlics on a leash plus dozens of dehydrated garlic products, many varieties of fresh garlic, hundreds of handsomely woven garlic braids as well as odorless garlic products.

While at the Gilroy Garlic Festival I met a lady named Anita Miramontez, who was 80 years old but actually looked about 55. She had nary a wrinkle that I could tell, and some of the smoothest skin I've ever seen. She lives in Guadalajara, Mexico, but had come up to visit the festival with some of her relatives. I asked her how she managed to retain her youthfulness. She blushed and replied that she owed her good looks to the garlic tonic she took every morning and evening.

When I asked for her recipe, she told me: Buy one quart of pure high-proof vodka. Peel one pound of garlic and pour the alcohol over it. Cover, set in a dark cool place for 30 days and do not disturb. All of the alcohol will eventually evaporate. The residue is strained and the garlic discarded. Each day make a wild sage tea by crushing one teaspoon of sage into one cup of boiling water. Cover and steep for 10 minutes. Add one teaspoon of the prepared garlic liquid to this tea and slowly sip it before breakfast and after dinner.

If you wish to attend this festival next year, contact:

Gilroy Garlic Festival Association, Inc.
P.O. Box 2311
Gilroy, CA 95021

Another garlic festival you might want to sample is:

Arizona's Own Garlic Festival
c/o Charles Onion
P.O. Box 2027
Campe Verde, AZ 86322

Garlic Doings in Europe

For some years now, the tiny village of Arleux, France, near the Belgian border, has produced over two million pounds of this pungent member of the lily family. That's enough garlic to take care of the total French domestic demand, some exports, and all of the scientific experiments conceived for the remainder of this decade and well into the next century.

So pleased with its agricultural contribution to world gastronomy and health is Arleux that it stages an all-out festival in celebration of the odoriferous white bulb every December. Stalls on Arleux's main street dispense garlicky dishes, including garlic soup, cheeses, sausages, and, of course, garlic bread. The festival reaches a glorious climax with a garlic ball in the town hall and the crowning of the elected "Garlic Queen."

For more information about this grand event, write:

French Government Tourist Office
625 Fifth Avenue
New York, NY
(212)-757-1125

The largest grower of culinary garlic in Europe is Colin Boswell of Mersley Farms on the Isle of Wight. His farms are situated in one of the most picturesque valleys on the island. The rich, red, alluvial soils are of a fine, porous sand and loam mixture, free-draining and able to hold the sun's heat. But the real merits of the Isle of Wight lie in its long hours of sunlight—just the thing for growing really flavorful garlic.

The garlic Colin cultivates is of French origin and has been developed by him through progressive selection to produce garlic that is fat and juicy while being both firm in texture and full of flavor. He now grows about 150 tons per year, all of which quickly vanishes into the cooking pots and frying pans of the United Kingdom. Colin supplies seed corms to those who wish to start growing their own, together with a leaflet with full instructions.

Each year, usually sometime in August, Colin and his dad, Martin, organize and run a garlic festival to rival the one in Arleux. The festival is held on a Sunday and about 37,000 visitors come with all the proceeds going to a worthwhile charity. There are marching bands with Scottish bagpipers dressed in woolen kilts, aerial acrobatics from daredevil flyers performing death-defying stunts, and motorcycle displays, not to mention the fun of an old-fashioned fair. For more details contact:

> Colin Boswell
> c/o Mersley Farms
> Newchurch, Isle of Wight
> PO 36 ONR Britain

CHAPTER EIGHT

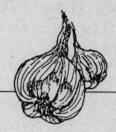

Garlic Recipes from Around the World

IN the last nineteen years I have traveled to almost three dozen countries to do research on botanical medicine. In the process of interviewing several hundred folk healers from many cultures, I picked up a number of recipes in addition to the medicinal remedies for specific health problems that I was after. I have gone through my large collections of such recipes and included here some of the very best ones that feature garlic.

Quite a few of these recipes not only taste good but are intended for healing purposes. In such instances they serve a dual function. The old adage is indeed true: food is your best medicine.

CAJUN-STYLE DISHES

Although Cajun cooking is unique to southern Louisiana, its origins may be found in France as far back as the 17th century, when a number of French Catholics emigrated to Nova Scotia in hopes of making a better life for themselves. Over a century later, when they were forced into exile by the British, many of them fled to South Louisiana and there found both the freedom and space to continue practicing their curious customs and strong religious beliefs.

In presenting the following Cajun dishes, it must be kept in mind that although they come from one of our southern states, they are more French Canadian in history and tradition than they are American. The ones selected here call for greater amounts of garlic than is usually found in most recipes, but those familiar with French cuisine know that garlic is an integral part of that dining experience, which has carried over into present day Cajun cooking.

NEW ORLEANS CHICKEN

Because of its four antibiotic herbs (garlic, onion, oregano, and thyme), this particular dish is especially healing during bouts with the common cold or flu. These ingredients boost the powers of the immune system in fighting infection.

1 5-pound stewing hen

½ cup olive oil

½ cup whole wheat flour

1¼ cups chopped onions

1 cup chopped celery (including leaves)

½ cup chopped green bell pepper

¾ cup diced garlic

10 button mushrooms

2 cups diced tomatoes

1 tbsp. finely diced jalapeños

½ cup tomato paste

1 tsp. crushed oregano

1½ tsp. dry thyme

1 tsp. basil

1 cup dry red wine

4 cups chicken stock

Salt to taste

Cut the hen into serving size pieces. Some of the larger pieces like the breasts may be cut into two pieces. In a two-gallon dutch oven, heat the oil over medium high heat. Add the flour and, using a wire whisk, stir constantly until golden brown roux is achieved. When browned add the onions, celery, bell pepper, garlic, mushrooms, tomatoes, and jalapeños. Sauté 5 to 10 minutes or until the vegetables are wilted. Then add the chicken and blend well. Continue cooking an additional three minutes. Next add the tomato paste, oregano, and thyme and blend well. Add the wine and chicken stock, a little at a time, stirring constantly until all is incorporated. Bring to a low boil and reduce to simmer. Cover and cook, stirring occasionally, about one hour. Add small amounts of chicken stock should the mixture become too thick. Season to taste with salt and continue cooking until the chicken is tender. Serve over brown or wild rice. Serves six.

CHICKEN PAELLA

This one dish has influenced Cajun cooking more than any other. Not only was it the forefather of present-day Louisiana jambalaya, it was the hearty dish that kept many Cajun families alive during the Great Depression and other hard economic times.

1 3-pound fryer chicken

½ cup olive oil

½ cup diced onions

½ cup diced celery (leaves intact)

¼ cup diced red bell pepper (seeds intact)

¼ cup diced green bell pepper (seeds intact)

½ cup diced green onions

½ cup diced garlic

½ cup sliced mushrooms

1 cup cooked black eyed peas

1 cup diced tomatoes

3 cups long grain rice

4 cups chicken stock (homemade or canned)

2 tsps. dried thyme

1 tsp. dried sweet basil

Salt (optional)

Lime juice

Cut the chicken into serving pieces and rub them well with the lime juice and optional salt. Set them aside. In a four-quart dutch oven, heat the olive oil over a medium high heat. Brown the chicken thoroughly on both sides, doing just a few pieces at a time. Remove them and keep warm. In the same oil add the onions, celery, both kinds of bell pepper, green onions, garlic, mushrooms, black eyed peas and tomatoes. Sauté 3 to 5 minutes or until these vegetables and spices are wilted. Then add the rice and stir fry into the vegetables for an additional 3 to 5 minutes. Next add the chicken stock, thyme, and basil. Season to taste using some more salt and lime juice, if necessary. Bring everything to a low boil and cook for slightly under five minutes, stirring occasionally. Finally, add the chicken, blend well into the rice and vegetable mixture, and reduce the heat to the lowest setting possible. Cover the pot with a lid and permit the rice to cook for 30 to 45 minutes, stirring at fifteen minute intervals. Serves six.

BAKED RIVER CATFISH

One of the most prevalent aspects of the Southern Louisiana land-scape is water. Everywhere you look there are bayous, swamps, bays, rivers, and lakes, not to mention the Gulf of Mexico. Each area features its own variety of fish or shellfish. From the rivers, fishermen pull tons of catfish, which enjoys a popularity in Louisiana unlike any other state.

FOR THE SAUCE:

¼ cup melted creamery butter

1 cup chopped onion

1 cup chopped celery (leaves intact)

½ cup chopped green bell pepper (seeds intact)

½ cup diced garlic

2 whole bay leaves

2 8-ounce cans tomato sauce

1 cup fish stock (homemade or canned)

½ tsp. brown sugar

⅛ tsp. dry thyme

⅛ tsp. dry sweet basil

1 cup chopped green onions

1 cup chopped parsley

Salt to taste

In a two-quart heavy saucepan, melt the butter over medium high heat. Sauté the onions, celery, bell pepper, garlic, and bay leaves until the vegetables are wilted, about 3 to 5 minutes. Then add the tomato sauce and fish stock, bring to a low boil, reduce to simmer and cook half an hour, stirring occasionally. Add the sugar, thyme, basil, green onions, and parsley. Continue to cook 10 additional minutes and season to taste with salt. Remove from the heat and set aside.

FOR THE FISH

4 catfish fillets

1 cup small shrimp, peeled and deveined

Lime juice

4 cups cooked white rice

¼ cup chopped parsley

Preheat the oven to 375° F. (190° C.). Place the catfish fillets in an ovenproof casserole large enough to hold the four fillets. Spread the shrimp evenly over the top of the fillets. Sprinkle with lime juice. Spoon on the prepared sauce until the catfish and shrimp are thoroughly covered. Place the covered baking dish in the oven and cook for half an hour or until the fish appears to be done. Put a mound of hot cooked rice in the center of each serving plate. Serve the river catfish on top of the white rice and garnish with chopped parsley. This dish can also be served over pasta. Serves six.

SPECTACULAR LUNCHEONS ON THE MEDITERRANEAN

Mediterranean food is not only delicious, but it is good for your health. Wild herbs blend with the earthy flavors of garlic, lentils, and garbanzo beans. Fresh, crisp vegetables contrast with the special tang of tahini—a paste made from olive oil and toasted sesame seeds.

Today doctors and nutritionists are encouraging patients who suffer from hypertension, coronary heart disease, diabetes, or simple overweight, to switch to a Mediterranean diet.

TACO FROM MOROCCO (PITA BREAD WITH FALAFELS)

1 piece of pita bread

2 to 3 falafels (see accompanying recipe)

¼ to ½ cup alfalfa sprouts

⅛ to ¼ cup chopped tomatoes

1 tbsp. sliced green onion

1 tsp. minced garlic

1 to 2 tbsps. tahini dressing (see accompanying recipe)

Many supermarkets and health food stores carry pita bread and tahini. Prepare the falafels and tahini dressing according to the accompanying recipes. Place the falafels in the bottom of the pita bread. Add the sprouts, tomatoes, green onions, and garlic. Drizzle with tahini dressing and eat. Serves one person.

FALAFELS

3 cups cooked chickpeas
  (garbanzo beans)
¼ cup liquid from the
  cooked chickpeas
1 small onion, finely
  chopped
2 garlic cloves, finely
  minced
4 tbsps. chopped fresh
  parsley

¼ cup sesame seeds
¼ tsp. each: sweet basil,
  tarragon, marjoram
1 tsp. cumin
1 tsp. chili powder
¼ cup lime juice
¼ to ¾ cup wheat germ

Place the chickpeas and their liquid into a blender and puree. Put the bean mixture in a large bowl and add all other ingredients except the wheat germ. Mix well. Stir in just enough wheat germ so that the mixture will hold together. With the hands, roll this mixture into balls about 1½ inches in diameter. Arrange them on a cookie sheet and bake in a preheated oven at 400° F. (204° C.) for half an hour, turning occasionally to brown evenly on all sides. Serve in pita bread or as an appetizer with tahini dressing. Serves eight to ten.

TAHINI DRESSING

1 cup tahini	2 tbsps. lime juice
½ cup water	4 cloves fresh garlic, crushed
½ cup plain yogurt	

Blend everything in a blender until smooth. Makes 2 cups.

ATHENS TOMATO LENTIL SOUP

After visiting the ancient ruins of the Parthenon on the Acropolis, I chanced to dine at a quaint little Greek bistro in an older section of Athens. They served this memorable soup.

8 ounces dry lentils	1 tsp. dried marjoram
4 cups water	3 garlic cloves, finely minced
1 medium onion, chopped	
3 potatoes, cubed	1½ cups cooked chopped tomatoes
2 to 3 carrots, sliced	
1 bay leaf	½ cup chopped spinach
1 to 2 tsps. dried sweet basil	Salt to taste

Rinse the lentils and place in a 5- to 6-quart pot with water, onions, potatoes, carrots and the seasonings. Bring to a boil. Lower heat and let it simmer, covered for an hour or until the lentils are very soft and the vegetables are tender. Then add the tomatoes and simmer for fifteen minutes. Add the spinach and cook until just wilted. Salt to taste. A dash of lime juice adds zest to an already great-tasting soup. If too thick, add tomato juice or water. Serves four to six.

HUMMOUS

1 can (15 ounces) of
chickpeas, including
liquid

¼ cup tahini or sesame
paste

2 tbsps. lemon juice

2 tbsps. lime juice

1 tbsp. orange juice

3 large garlic cloves, cut
into thirds

½ tsp. cumin

Salt to taste

Chopped fresh parsley to
garnish

Drain the chickpeas, reserving their liquid. Put them into a blender or food processor. Add the tahini, citrus juices, garlic, cumin, and ¼ cup of chickpea liquid. Blend or process slowly, adding more chickpea liquid if required, until the entire mixture has become smooth and has the consistency of thick pancake batter. Season to taste with salt. Sprinkle with chopped parsley and serve with pita triangles.

GREEK SALAD WITH LEMON-GARLIC DRESSING

½ head iceberg lettuce, torn
into bite-size pieces

1 bunch romaine lettuce or
green leaf lettuce, torn
into bite-size pieces

1 cucumber, thinly sliced

3 green onions with tops,
thinly sliced

2 garlic cloves, peeled and
thinly sliced on a
diagonal

3 red radishes, sliced

3 white radishes, sliced

3 black radishes, sliced

3 tomatoes, cut into eight
wedges each

12 to 18 Greek or black
olives

Feta cheese, crumbled, to
garnish

Lemon-Garlic Dressing
(recipe to follow)

Arrange the greens in the center of a large platter. Cover the greens with a row of sliced cucumbers. Sprinkle with sliced green onions and garlic, surround them with the sliced radishes, and encircle the edge of the platter with tomato wedges. Garnish with the olives and sprinkle with feta cheese. Serve with Lemon-Garlic Dressing. Serves six to eight.

LEMON-GARLIC DRESSING

½ cup pure virgin olive oil

¼ cup lemon juice

¼ cup lime juice

2 to 3 garlic cloves, peeled, halved, and speared on toothpick

Salt to taste

In a small bowl, combine the oil, citrus juices, and salt. Drop in the garlic spears. Let stand at room temperature for an hour or more. Remove the garlic just prior to serving. Makes about one cup.

A LITTLE BIT OF ITALIA

When I was in Italy in 1980, I quickly discerned from the breath of just about everyone whom I encountered that Italians love garlic! This, along with their liberal use of olive oil and enthusiasm for vegetables may explain their over-all good health.

STUFFED MUSHROOMS WITH GARLIC AND PARSLEY

12 large fresh mushrooms

1 tbsp. finely chopped lemon peel

1 tbsp. finely chopped lime peel

2 tbsps. fresh lemon juice, strained

2 tbsps. fresh lime juice, strained

Salt to taste

2 tbsps. olive oil

4 garlic cloves, finely chopped

1 cup chopped fresh parsley

6 tbsps. fresh bread crumbs

Carefully remove the stems from the mushrooms. To clean the mushrooms, wipe each one of them with a damp towel. Preheat the oven to 375° F. (190° C.). Arrange the mushrooms on a tray, concave side up, and lightly sprinkle each mushroom cap with lemon and lime juice and the chopped peels of both. Season with salt to taste. Heat the oil in a skillet over a medium-high heat, then add the garlic, and sauté about two minutes. Be sure that the garlic doesn't brown. Remove from the heat and add the parsley and bread crumbs. Toss or still well. Fill each mushroom cap with the filling mixture. Handling carefully, arrange the filled mushrooms on an oiled cookie sheet, with the filling side turned up. Bake for 15 minutes, watching carefully for the last few minutes of baking; the mushroom caps should stay firm. Serves eight.

ITALIAN PASTA SAUCE

2 quarts canned tomatoes

3 6-ounce cans tomato paste

1 green pepper, chopped

2 tbsps. each oregano and
   sweet basil

8 garlic cloves, minced

1 tsp. onion powder

1 bay leaf

2 tsp. dark honey

1 tsp. lime juice

Combine all of the ingredients in a large pan. Bring to a gentle simmer over medium heat. Let simmer at least one hour. The longer the sauce simmers, the better the flavor. When cooking is completed, remove the bay leaf. This sauce keeps for long periods in the freezer. Makes 2½ quarts, or enough for 10 servings.

PESTO SAUCE

6 large garlic cloves

1 packed cup fresh parsley,
   tough stems removed

1 packed cup basil leaves,
   tough stems removed

1 cup olive oil

½ cup grated imported
   Parmesan cheese

Place the garlic, parsley, and basil in a blender and mix until all the ingredients are finely chopped. Then add the pure virgin olive oil and blend for 20 seconds. Add the grated cheese and blend for another 15 seconds. This recipe makes about 1½ cups. The extra sauce can be stored in the refrigerator for up to three weeks or kept in the freezer for about two months. Be sure that the basil leaves and parsley are submerged in the olive oil. Warm to room temperature before using.

FRENCH FINESSE IN FOOD PREPARATION

The "French paradox" is hard for medical researchers to explain. The French diet abounds in butter, cheese, foie gras (the fattened livers of ducks and geese), creamy sauces, and very rich pastries—all of which are very high in fat—yet the French have less than half the heart disease of the U.S. They also smoke more than we do and don't exercise much.

In the last year or so, *The New York Times*, "60 Minutes," *Newsweek* magazine, *USA Today*, the *Journal of Applied Cardiology*, and various monthly health and wellness newsletters have discussed this dietary phenomenon at some length. Several important factors have emerged which may account for this paradox. First of all, the French drink more red wine with their heavy, artery-clogging meals, and wine has been shown to possess special cholesterol-altering effects which can prevent hardening of the arteries. Second, the French use a lot of garlic, and garlic has been found repeatedly to lower "bad" serum cholesterol and the triglycerides which can bring on heart disease. Third, the French, as a rule, usually take an hour or more to enjoy their meals; they don't gulp their food in a hurried rush as so many of us are apt to do. Finally, in spite of their rich diets, they generally avoid snacking on junk foods, which tend to be high in altered or hyrdrogenated fats.

The following recipes from Southern France certainly aren't intended for weight watchers but for those who "live to eat" and are thin enough or healthy enough to tolerate rich foods. Every tasty, high-fat recipe presented here calls for plenty of garlic to keep the heart reasonably healthy and free of congestive failure while you indulge in scrumptious French-style meals.

VERY GARLICKY MASHED POTATOES

4 cups peeled cut up white potatoes

1 cup peeled garlic cloves

½ cup milk

2 tbsps. sweet butter

Chopped fresh parsley

Salt and pepper to taste

Simmer the potatoes, covered with salted water, until tender. Drain and mash with the butter. While the potatoes cook, heat the garlic and milk in a medium saucepan. Simmer until the garlic is soft, or for about half an hour. Puree in a blender. Then whisk the puree into the mashed potato. Season with salt and pepper to taste. Garnish with chopped parsley.

CHICKEN LIVERS WITH SPINACH NOODLES

¾ lb. chicken livers

2 tbsps. pure virgin olive oil

½ lb. thinly sliced mushrooms

Salt to taste

2 tbsps. finely chopped shallots

4 tbsps. chopped garlic

1 cup canned crushed tomatoes

4 ripe plum tomatoes, cored and cut into ½-inch cubes

2 tbsps. chopped fresh basil

1 cup flour for dredging

3 tbsps. olive oil

¾ lb. green spinach noodles

Cut the livers in half. Pick over and discard any tough connecting membranes. Set aside. Heat the olive oil in a skillet over medium heat. When crackling hot, add the mushrooms and salt. Cook, stirring often, until the mushrooms are lightly browned. Then add the shallots and garlic and cook, stirring, until they become limp. Make sure you don't brown the garlic. Next add the crushed tomatoes, cubed tomatoes, basil, and salt. Bring everything to a boil and simmer 5 minutes. Set aside. In the meantime, put the flour in a flat dish. Add some salt, and blend together well. Add the livers and stir thoroughly to coat them. Remove them and shake off the excess flour.

Heat the olive oil in a large skillet over a medium-high heat. Add the livers a handful at a time and cook, turning as necessary so they brown evenly and are crisp, for about 3 minutes. Then transfer them with a slotted spoon to the mushroom mixture. Cook the noodles to the desired doneness. Drain them, but reserve ¼ cup of the liquid. Return them to the pot, add the liver-mushroom mixture and the cooking liquid. Over a medium heat blend and toss gently but thoroughly. Serves four.

HEARTY BEEF STEW FROM LE VACCARÈS

3 cups dry red wine

3 cups beef stock or canned low-salt broth

10 garlic cloves, chopped

1 onion, chopped

3 carrots, chopped

¼ cup olive oil

½ cup brandy

¼ cup red wine vinegar

Bouquet garni (6 thyme sprigs, 6 parsley stems, 2 bay leaves)

4 lbs. boneless beef chuck, cut into 1-inch pieces

1 cup whole garlic cloves, peeled

3 anchovy fillets, chopped

1 tbsp. drained capers

Cooked rice

Combine the wine, stock, 5 chopped garlic cloves, ½ of the chopped onion, carrots, 2 tbsps. of the olive oil, the brandy, vinegar and bouquet garni in a bowl. Add the beef. Cover with plastic wrap and refrigerate overnight. Heat the remaining 2 tbsps. of oil in a large, heavy pot over medium heat. Add the remaining chopped garlic and onion and saute until golden, for about 5 minutes. Add the beef, its marinade, and the whole garlic cloves. Cover and simmer until the beef is tender, for about two hours.

Drain the cooking liquid from the beef into a large, heavy saucepan. Discard the bouquet garni. Degrease the liquid. Boil until it's reduced to only two cups, for about an hour. Pour this sauce over the meat. Rewarm the stew over a medium fire. Stir in the anchovies and capers. Simmer ten minutes. Serve over brown or wild rice, noodles, or boiled potatoes. Serves six to eight.

SOUTH OF THE BORDER

Many Mexican dishes of today are a result of the blending of indigenous Indian cultures and the Spaniards who conquered them. The recipes that follow reflect an amalgamation of tastes from the Old World as well as the New.

TOLUCA REFRIED BLACK BEANS

Beans are one of the best foods to keep serum cholesterol and triglyceride levels normal, maintain proper sugar metabolism, and help bowel activity to stay regular.

1 cup dry black beans, rinsed and soaked overnight

2 tbsps. olive oil

4 large cloves garlic, finely minced

1 tbsp. dried or minced fresh epazote

Salt to taste

Drain beans and put into a large cooking pot with enough water to cover. Bring to simmer, cover, and cook 1½ hours. Don't drain. Heat the oil in a skillet and sauté the garlic and epazote. Add part of the cooked beans along with some bean stock and mash with the back of a thick wooden ladle. Repeat with the rest of the beans, keeping the consistency rather soupy. Season with salt. Heat beans several minutes until thoroughly warmed. Serves four.

CUERNAVACA SALSA VERDE

12 tomatillos, husked and rinsed

4 large cloves garlic

½ cup loosely packed cilantro leaves

1 tbsp. olive oil

1 tbsp. apple cider vinegar

1 jalapeño pepper, stemmed and deseeded

Salt to taste

Simmer the tomatillos in enough water to cover for 15 minutes. Remove from water. Combine with the remaining ingredients in a blender or food processor. Blend to the desired consistency. Then season with salt. Makes about 1½ cups.

CAMPECHE SALSA FRESCA

dash of commercial hot pepper sauce

1 large tomato, chopped

1 medium avocado, chopped

1 tbsp. minced fresh cilantro

1 tbsp. fresh lime juice

4 cloves garlic, minced

½ tsp. salt

Combine all of the ingredients and mix well in a food processor. Yields about two cups of mild sauce.

SALSA DE AGUACATE

3 tomatillos, husked and rinsed

2 cups water

2 large ripe avocados, peeled, pits removed, chopped

2 habanero chiles, stems and seeds removed, chopped

4 cloves garlic

Combine the tomatillos and water and boil until they are soft, about 12 minutes. Drain and discard the water. Puree all the ingredients in a blender or food processor, adding a little water if needed to make the salsa smooth and creamy. Serve with tostadas. Yields 2 cups of hot salsa.

VERACRUZ GUACAMOLE

3 small heads (not cloves) fresh garlic

1 dark-green, ripe avocado

1 package (3 oz.) Philadelphia cream cheese, softened

3 tbsps. sour cream

1 tbsp. lime juice

1 tbsp. sour orange juice

1 tbsp. lemon juice

½ tsp. salt

Place the whole heads of garlic into a baking dish, drizzle with some olive oil and roast in a 350° F. (177° C.) oven for an hour. When cool, gently separate the cloves and squeeze the garlic out into a wooden bowl. Peel and pit the avocado, add it to the garlic along with the remaining ingredients. Mash with the back of a heavy wooden spoon until smooth in consistency. Serve with low-salt corn or taco chips or else use as a topping for other Mexican dishes. Makes about 1¼ cups.

CHICKEN ITZA GARLIC-LIME SOUP

This delicate soup from the Yucatan is very popular all over Mexico. This particular recipe is especially good for sinusitis, allergies, asthma, hay fever, common cold, and influenza.

3 corn tortillas, cut in strips

Corn oil for frying

2 chicken breasts

5 cloves garlic, chopped

6 black peppercorns

1 2-inch stick cinnamon

8 whole allspice

Small handful raisins

1 tbsp. chopped fresh oregano

4 cups chicken broth

1 tomato, peeled and chopped

6 tbsps. lime juice

1 green Mexican chile, roasted, peeled, stems and seeds removed, chopped

5 lime slices

Chopped cilantro for garnish

Fry the tortilla strips in 360° F. (182° C.) corn oil until crisp. Remove, drain on paper towels, and keep warm. Place the chicken, garlic, peppercorns, cinnamon, allspice, raisins, orgeano, and broth in a pot. Bring to a rapid boil, then reduce the heat to medium, and simmer, covered, for half an hour. Let the chicken cool in the stock. Then shred the meat with your fingers or two forks. Strain the broth and add just enough water to make a quart of liquid. Reheat the broth with the tomato, lime juice, and chile. Add the chicken and simmer until the chicken is hot. To serve, place some of the tortilla chips in the bottom of a soup bowl, add the soup, garnish with a slice of lime, and serve. Serves about five.

ACAPULCO AVOCADO BISQUE

2 bunches spinach, heated
    until just wilted but not
    overcooked
2 medium avocados
7 cloves fresh garlic

1 cup cream
1 cup chicken broth
1 tbsp. butter
1 tsp. salt

Place everything in a blender and mix for one minute until creamy smooth. Then pour into a saucepan and cover. Heat on medium until hot, but don't boil. Serve at once. Makes a quart.

OAXACA GARLIC TORTILLA SOPA (SOUP)

18 cloves fresh garlic
1¼ cups water
2 cans (11 oz. each) chicken
    broth
Juice of 2 limes
2 corn tortillas, cut into
    ½-inch pieces

3 egg yolks
Dash of paprika
Dash of Tabasco sauce
Pinch of cumin
Pinch of coriander

Peel the garlic, then mix the garlic and water in a blender until well combined. Place this in a two-quart saucepan with the broth and lime juice. Simmer for half an hour. Add the tortillas and cook another ten minutes. Remove from the stove and cool until luke-warm. Slowly add the egg yolks, stirring constantly with a wire whisk. Reheat and add the paprika, cumin, coriander, and Tabasco. Makes four hearty servings.

The Beautiful Cuisine of Mysterious China

Food in all its aspects has, since the birth of Chinese civilization, been a cornerstone of the national culture. In no other country has the preparation, preservation, cooking, cultivation, and serving of food taken such a dominant role. China's very history revolves around the table and the kitchen.

Intertwined with the love of good food is the ancient basic philosophy of China, a belief in harmony, the balance of nature, the duality of existence, the blending of contrasts. Yin and yang, the two elements, are as significant in the Chinese kitchen as they are in the temple. In the wok, hot pot, or steamer, yin and yang combine and complement each other. Sweet contrasts with sour. The two basics of stir-frying—ginger and green onions or ginger and garlic—are yang and yin. Crunchy sea salt goes with Sichuan peppercorns, steamed chicken goes with stir-fried fresh greens, the yang of fiery chilies goes with the gentle yin of sugar.

When I went to China in 1980 I made sure to collect every good recipe I could find. The dishes that follow were part of those efforts and reflect the generous use of garlic by the earth's oldest and, some say, most ingenious people.

SMOKED DUCK WITH TENDER GINGER

1 whole breast of a smoked duck

12 slices young fresh ginger

1 to 2 fresh red chilies

2 green onions

3 cloves garlic

2 tbsps. oil for frying

1 tsp. brown sugar

SEASONING

2 tbsps. light soy sauce

1 tbsp. hot bean paste

2½ tsps. sugar

2 tsps. rice vinegar

Don't skin the duck, but cut the breast into thin slices, then stack several slices on top of each other and cut them into narrow shreds. Cut the ginger, chilies, and green onions into shreds and slice the garlic. Heat the oil in a wok to the smoking point and stir-fry the duck until crisp on the edges. Remove and set aside. Stir-fry the vegetables and garlic together for about 2 minutes, then add the seasoning ingredients and stir-fry together for another 30 seconds. Return the duck meat and continue to stir-fry over high heat until all ingredients are well mixed. Stir in the brown vinegar and serve.

SPECIAL BRAISED ROCK CARP

1 one-pound rock carp or
    other meaty white fresh-
    water fish

6 oz. yam

3 green onions

3 slices fresh ginger

4 cloves garlic

2 tbsps. lard

1 tbsp. rice wine or dry
    sherry

1 tbsp. hot bean paste

1 tbsp. sugar

1 tbsp. brown vinegar

1 tbsp. rice wine

1 tbsp. light soy sauce

Pinch of kelp

SAUCE

2 cups water

Clean the fish and make several diagonal slashes across each side. Peel and finely dice the yam. Chop the green onions, ginger and garlic finely. In a wok, sauté the yam in the lard for about 3 minutes until lightly colored, then place in the bottom of a casserole dish. Add the fish to the wok, sauté on both sides until lightly colored and place on top of the yam. Lightly fry the green onions, ginger and garlic in the lard and add to the casserole with the pre-mixed sauce ingredients. Bring to a rapid boil, skim any froth and residue from the surface and reduce the heat. Simmer very gently, partially covered, until the fish is tender and the stock reduced to a thick layer over the fish. Serves six.

TWICE-COOKED BEEF

2 lbs. beef bottom round

3 tbsps. peanut oil

3 pieces star anise

2 pieces dried tangerine peel

1 green onion

8 slices fresh ginger

5 cloves garlic

1 tsp. Sichuan peppercorns

3 tbsps. rice wine or dry sherry

½ cup light soy sauce

3 tbsps. dark soy sauce

2 tbsps. brown bean sauce

1 tbsp. sugar

Kelp to taste

2 tsps. cornstarch

1 tsp. sesame oil

Cut the beef into thick slices, then into square pieces. In a wok, heat the oil to the smoking point and fry the beef in several batches until well colored. Lift out and set aside. Drain off most of the oil. Stir-fry the star anise, peel, whole onion, ginger, garlic, and peppercorns for 3 minutes. Add the wine and soy sauces and simmer for 5 minutes. Discard the star anise, green onion, ginger and garlic, then add the beef slices, bean sauce, and sugar. Cover with water. Bring to a boil, then reduce the heat to very low and simmer, covered, for about 3 hours. Season the sauce with kelp and thicken with cornstarch mixed with cold water. Sprinkle with the sesame oil and serve at once. Serves six.

GOLDEN RICE WITH BOK CHOY

4 cups freshly cooked white
    rice (about 1½ cups
    raw rice)

4 cloves garlic

3 oz. peeled shrimp

2 chicken livers

5 medium eggs

1 tbsp. water

pinch of salt

¼ cup vegetable oil

1 tsp. sesame oil

6 stalks bok choy or other
    Chinese green vegetable

½ cup water

SEASONING

2 tbsps. light soy sauce

1 tsp. salt

1 tsp. sugar

⅓ tsp. white pepper

Spread the cooked rice on a tray to cool. Very finely chop the garlic, then dice the shrimp and chicken livers. Beat the eggs lightly in a small bowl, adding 1 tbsp. water and a pinch of salt.

Heat half the vegetable oil in a wok and stir-fry the garlic for half a minute. Add the shrimp and chicken livers and stir-fry until they change color and begin to firm up. Add the rice and stir-fry until warmed through. Add the seasoning ingredients and mix in well. Pour in the beaten eggs and continue to stir-fry over low heat until the eggs are lightly cooked.

Pile into a heated plate and shape into a flat mound. Keep warm. Heat the remaining vegetable oil in the wok and add the sesame oil. Put in the bok choy and stir-fry briefly, then add the water, cover and cook until the vegetables are tender. Arrange around the rice and serve.

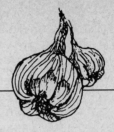

Appendix

THE latest garlic research information and practical applications for its use, are published in every other issue of an alternative health care quarterly entitled FOLK MEDICINE JOURNAL. John Heinerman, Ph.D., the author of this book, is the editor-in-chief, with Linda Steele as the managing editor. Subscription rates are $30 per year in North America and $35 overseas. When subscribing, please make your check out to Dr. John Heinerman and send it to:

Anthropological Research Center
P.O. Box 11471
Salt Lake City, UT 84147

For the Chinese perspective on garlic, three small booklets by a medical researcher and nutritionist may be helpful. They are *Garlic For Health* and *Garlic Research Update* by Benjamin Lau, M.D., Ph.D., and *Garlic in Nutrition and Medicine* by Robert I-San Lin, Ph.D. They are free provided the necessary postage of $5.00 for shipping and handling is sent *in stamps* (not check or cash). Send postage stamps and your name, address, zip code, and telephone number to:

> Garlic Information Center
> 3493 Augusta Dr.
> Ijamsville, MD 21754
> 1-800-233-6550

To learn more about the therapeutic benefits of garlic from a medicinal as well as nutritional perspective, a special correspondence course is available from a fully approved educational institution. The International University For Nutrition Education (IUNE) is authorized by the State of California Department of Education Private Postsecondary Education Division as a degree granting institution. Established in 1977 as a non-profit university, IUNE offers Baccalaureate, Masters, and Doctor of Philosophy degrees in Clinical Nutrition and Botanical Medicine as well as Continuing Education programs. For further information, contact:

> Jacob Swilling, Ph.D., DPN
> President
> IUNE
> 1161-A Bay Boulevard
> Chula Vista, CA 91911
> (619) 424-7590

A monthly senior citizens' newspaper, now in its fourth year of publication and edited by the author of this book, frequently features practical health tips, recipes, and assorted handicrafts involving garlic. To receive a year's subscription, send a check for $10 made out to Senior Prime Times to the following address:

Senior Prime Times
190 West 2950 South
Salt Lake City, UT 84115
(801) 485-5511
1-800-848-1016

Readers may be interested in ordering one of my previously published works related to garlic. It is entitled *The Complete Book of Spices* and may be obtained from Keats Publishing, Inc., Box 876, New Canaan, CT 06840-0876.

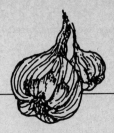

Index